Practical Weight Management in Dogs and Cats

Practical Weight Management in Dogs and Cats

Edited by

Todd L. Towell
DVM, MS, DACVIM

⊛WILEY-BLACKWELL

A John Wiley & Sons, Inc., Publication

Registered office: John Wiley & Sons Ltd, The Atrium, Southern Gate, Chichester, West Sussex, PO19 8SQ, UK

Editorial offices: 2121 State Avenue, Ames, Iowa 50014-8300, USA
The Atrium, Southern Gate, Chichester, West Sussex, PO19 8SQ, UK
9600 Garsington Road, Oxford, OX4 2DQ, UK

For details of our global editorial offices, for customer services and for information about how to apply for permission to reuse the copyright material in this book please see our website at www.wiley.com/wiley-blackwell.

Library of Congress Cataloging-in-Publication Data
Practical weight management in dogs and cats / edited by Todd L. Towell.
      p. ; cm.
    Includes bibliographical references and index.
    ISBN 978-0-8138-0956-4 (pbk. : alk. paper)
    1. Cats–Diseases–Diet therapy.   2. Dogs–Diseases–Diet therapy.   3. Cats–Exercise.
4. Dogs–Exercise.   5. Obesity in animals.   I. Towell, Todd L.
    [DNLM: 1. Obesity–therapy.   2. Obesity–veterinary.   3. Cats.   4. Dogs.
    SF 992.N88]
    SF985.P65 2011
    636.8'083–dc22

                                        2011007211

A catalogue record for this book is available from the British Library.
This book is published in the following electronic formats: ePDF 9780470960974; ePub 9780470960981; Mobi 9780470960998

Set in 10 on 12 pt Palatino by Toppan Best-set Premedia Limited

1   2011

Table of Contents

List of Contributors

P. Jane Armstrong, *DVM, MS, MBA, DACVIM*
Professor, Veterinary Internal Medicine
University of Minnesota College of Veterinary Medicine

Mark A. Brady, *DVM, DACVECC*
Veterinary Consultation Service
Hill's Pet Nutrition Inc.

Kara Burns, *MS, MEd, LVT*
Veterinary Technician Specialist
Hill's Pet Nutrition Inc.

Sharon Campbell, *DVM, MS, DACVIM*
Specialty Hospital Liaison
Pfizer Animal Health

S. Dru Forrester, *DVM, MS, DACVIM*
Associate Director, Scientific Communications
Hill's Pet Nutrition Inc.

Angela L. Lusby, *DVM, PhD, DACVN*
Clinical Instructor
University of Tennessee College of Veterinary Medicine

Denis J. Marcellin-Little, *DEDV, DACVS, DECVS, DACVSMR*
Professor, Orthopedics
North Carolina State University College of Veterinary Medicine

Rebecca L. Remillard, *PhD, DVM, DACVN*
Nutritionist
MSPCA Angell Animal Medical Center

Todd L. Towell, *DVM, MS, DACVIM*
Senior Manager, Scientific Communications
Hill's Pet Nutrition Inc.

Practical Weight Management in Dogs and Cats

Clinical Importance of Canine and Feline Obesity

P. Jane Armstrong, DVM, MS, MBA, DACVIM, and Angela L. Lusby, DVM, PhD, DACVN

Introduction

The last decade has seen a fundamental shift in our understanding of obesity. The discovery of hormones and cytokines generated by adipose tissue (termed adipokines) has expanded fat's traditional roles as an energy storage depot, insulator, and support for abdominal organs. Fat is now recognized as the most abundant source of hormones in the body, making it the largest endocrine organ. Additionally, macrophages in adipose tissue contribute to the release of numerous inflammatory cytokines and other adipokines into the blood. As a result, overweight and obese individuals reside in a state of chronic inflammation (Figure 1.1).

This knowledge has come on the heels of an epidemic of obesity in companion animals that parallels the global obesity epidemic in human patients. The combination of serious metabolic and health consequences of obesity and sheer number of obese pets should make canine and feline obesity a priority for veterinarians. Just as veterinarians have long provided routine infectious disease and dental prophylaxis, preventive health care also must focus on nutrition counseling. Informing pet owners about disease risk factors associated with obesity and recommending appropriate dietary intake for obesity prevention and weight loss should be integrated into most preventive care examinations.

Practical Weight Management in Dogs and Cats, First Edition. Edited by Todd L. Towell.
© 2011 John Wiley and Sons, Inc. Published 2011 by John Wiley & Sons, Inc.

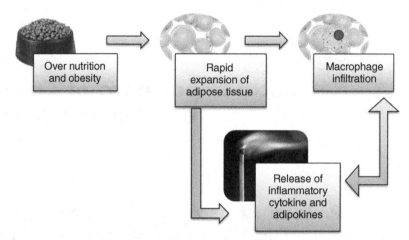

Figure 1.1. Relationship of obesity to chronic inflammation. In obese states, adipose tissue expands rapidly and adipocytes enlarge. This induces a state of local hypoxia and stress responses that recruit macrophages to adipose tissue. In the obese state, adipocytes also release cytokines, adipokines, and free fatty acids. These work locally and systemically to increase the inflammatory state within adipose tissue, liver, and muscle, and cause insulin resistance. Images from Fotolia.com.

Defining Obesity

Obesity is a disease in which excess body fat has accumulated such that health may be adversely affected. In human medicine, application of this definition is based on epidemiologic data that demonstrate increased morbidity and mortality risks with increasing body fat mass. Based on such data, criteria have been established for what constitutes "overweight" and "obese." To date, such objective criteria are not available for dogs and cats. Fat mass comprises about 15% to 20% of the body weight in dogs and cats in ideal body condition.[1–5] Pets are typically considered overweight at 10% to 20% above their ideal body weight and obese if their weight exceeds 20% to 30% more than ideal.[6,7]

One of the most difficult challenges in diagnosing obesity is determining ideal body weight and present fat mass. A patient's fat mass can be measured using a variety of methods. However, most involve some procedure or parameter that makes them unsuitable at present for routine clinical use. Because of its precision and relative ease of use, dual energy X-ray absorptiometry (DEXA) has become the standard tool for measuring body composition when performing clinical research in pet obesity. Unfortunately, access to DEXA equipment is generally limited to academic and corporate research facilities.

Similarity in shape among human patients permits the use of the body mass index (BMI), a number calculated as weight (kg) divided by height^2 (m). Similar semi-quantitative indices are not available for pets.

Because of the wide breed differences in body types, the equivalent of a BMI is unlikely to be developed for dogs. A BMI has been described for cats based on ribcage circumference and leg length measurements, but has not yet gained wide acceptance in clinical practice or research.[8] This may be partly because accurate measurements are difficult to make in an awake, active cat.

The standard method of semi-quantitatively assessing degree of adiposity in dogs and cats in a clinical setting is the use of a body condition scoring system. The advantage of assigning a body condition score (BCS) is that it provides more information than body weight, which often varies markedly, even within individuals of the same breed and gender. Veterinary clinicians and researchers most often use one of two semi-quantitative BCS systems (nine-point and five-point scales) that are based on visual and palpatory findings (Table 1.1).[4,9–12] It is important to keep in mind that these BCS systems were developed for use in healthy animals. For example, sick animals with conditions that lead to weight gain and marked muscle wasting (hyperadrenocorticism) are very difficult to score; therefore, simultaneous use of a muscle scoring system is recommended (Table 1.2).[13,14]

Prevalence of Obesity

The number of pets that are overweight or obese has reached epidemic proportions in the United States and other industrialized countries. Approximately 25% to 35% and 35% to 40% adult cats and dogs, respectively, are either overweight or obese.[15–17] Middle-aged neutered male cats and middle-aged spayed female dogs are at highest risk of becoming obese. Some purebred dogs also have higher obesity risks; these include Shetland Sheepdogs, Golden Retrievers, Dachshunds, Cocker Spaniels, Labrador Retrievers, Dalmatians, and Rottweilers.[17] Manx cats are more likely to become obese than other purebred cats. Not surprisingly, low activity level increases risk for weight gain in both species; in cats, apartment dwelling is associated with a higher risk. Obesity in dogs is associated with the number of meals and snacks fed, the feeding of table scraps, and the dog's presence when its owners prepare or eat their own meal.[16,17]

Veterinarians must proactively focus on obesity prevention. Wellness visits are the ideal time to regularly reassess body weight history and body condition score. The benefits of maintaining a pet in lean body condition, and the health risks that can accompany obesity, are important owner education topics. The veterinary visit for spaying/neutering is an important, but often neglected, opportunity to reassess feeding practices and discuss obesity issues with clients. Studies in cats have shown that neutering decreases metabolic rate by 25% to 33%.[18] Neutered animals, however, usually have increased fat mass. When

Table 1.1. Comparison of body condition scoring systems with body fat percentages.

5-point scale	9-point scale	% Body fat	Description
1	1	≤5	Emaciated: Ribs and bony prominences are visible from a distance. No palpable body fat. Obvious abdominal tuck and loss of muscle mass.
2	2	6–9	Very thin: Ribs and bony prominences visible. Minimal loss of muscle mass, but no palpable fat.
	3	10–14	Thin: Ribs easily palpable, tops of lumbar are visible. Obvious waist and abdominal tuck.
3	4	15–19	Lean: Ribs easily palpable, waist visible from above. Abdominal tuck present in dogs. Abdominal fat pad absent in cats.
	5	20–24	Ideal: Ribs palpable without excess fat covering. Waist and abdominal tuck present in dogs. Cats have a waist and a minimal abdominal fat pad.
4	6	25–29	Slightly overweight: Ribs have slight excess fat covering. Waist discernible from above, but not obvious. Abdominal tuck still present in dogs. Abdominal fat pad is apparent, but not obvious in cats.
	7	30–34	Overweight: Difficult to palpate ribs. Dogs: Fat deposits over lumbar area and tail base. Abdominal tuck may be present, but waist is absent. Cats: Moderate abdominal fat pad and rounding of the abdomen.
5	8	35–39	Obese: Ribs not palpable and abdomen may be rounded. Dogs: Heavy fat deposits over lumbar and base of tail. No abdominal tuck or waist. Cats: Prominent abdominal fat pad and lumbar fat deposits.
	9	40–45+	Morbidly obese: Dogs: Large fat deposits over thorax, tail base, and spine, with abdominal distension. Cats: Heavy fat deposits over lumbar area, face, and limbs. Large abdominal fat pad and rounded abdomen.

Adapted from Lusby A, Kirk C. 2008. Obesity. *Kirk's Current Veterinary Therapy XIV*. St. Louis: Saunders Elsevier.

energy expenditure is expressed on a lean mass basis, no difference in metabolic rate is noted between neutered and entire individuals (REF). An alternative explanation for the effect of neutering on obesity is an alteration in feeding behavior leading to increased food intake and decreased activity, without a corresponding decrease in energy intake.

Table 1.2. Muscle scoring system.

Score	Fat mass	Muscle mass
0	Absence of palpable subcutaneous fat over the ribs or the abdominal region	Severe muscle wasting as evidenced by pronounced decreased muscle mass palpable over the scapulae, skull, or wings of the ilia
1	Decreased amounts of palpable subcutaneous fat of the ribs or the abdominal region	Moderate muscle wasting as evidenced by clearly discernible decreased muscle mass palpable over the scapulae, skull, or wings of the ilia
2	Normal amounts of palpable subcutaneous fat over the ribs or the abdominal region	Mild muscle wasting as evidenced by slight but discernible decreased muscle mass palpable over the scapulae, skull, or wings of the ilia
3	Increased amounts of palpable subcutaneous fat over the ribs or the abdominal region	Normal muscle mass palpable over the scapulae, skull, or wings of the ilia

Adapted from Michel KE, Sorenmo K, Shofer FS. 2004. Evaluation of body condition and weight loss in dogs presented to a veterinary oncology service. *Journal of Veterinary Internal Medicine* 18:692–695.

Health Risks of Obesity

Diseases associated with obesity in human patients include hypertension, coronary heart disease, dyslipidemias, and type-2 diabetes mellitus (these conditions form the components of so-called metabolic syndrome), as well as certain cancers (breast, ovarian, and prostate), osteoarthritis, respiratory disease such as asthma, and reproductive disorders.[19-22] Studies investigating overweight or obese dogs and cats have identified many of the same chronic health problems observed in obese humans.

Obesity in companion animals is a serious medical concern, resulting in a shorter life span and greater disease morbidity. Dietary restriction can increase longevity in other species, and a landmark prospective study in Labrador Retrievers yielded the same result.[23] In this study, 24 pairs of dogs were enrolled as puppies with one dog in each pair randomly assigned to consume food *ad libitum*. The paired dog was fed 75% of the amount consumed by its counterpart. In the energy-restricted group, the mean body condition score was 4.5/9 compared to 6.8/9 in the *ad libitum* feeding group. Causes of death did not differ between the two groups, but life span was increased by 1.8 years in the energy-restricted group (median 13 years vs. 11.2 years). Dogs in the lean body condition group also had reduced risk of hip dysplasia and osteoarthritis and improved glucose tolerance.

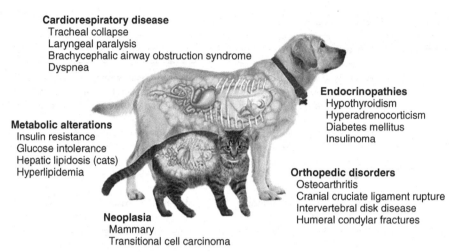

Cardiorespiratory disease
Tracheal collapse
Laryngeal paralysis
Brachycephalic airway obstruction syndrome
Dyspnea

Endocrinopathies
Hypothyroidism
Hyperadrenocorticism
Diabetes mellitus
Insulinoma

Metabolic alterations
Insulin resistance
Glucose intolerance
Hepatic lipidosis (cats)
Hyperlipidemia

Orthopedic disorders
Osteoarthritis
Cranial cruciate ligament rupture
Intervertebral disk disease
Humeral condylar fractures

Neoplasia
Mammary
Transitional cell carcinoma

Figure 1.2. Diseases associated with obesity in dogs and cats. Courtesy Hill's Pet Nutrition, Inc.

In cats, diabetes mellitus, neoplasia, dental disease, dermatologic diseases, and lower urinary tract problems have been associated with obesity.[24] In dogs, obesity has been linked with insulin resistance, pancreatitis, cruciate ligament rupture, lower urinary tract disease, oral disease, neoplasia (mammary tumors, transitional cell carcinoma), abnormalities in circulating lipid profiles, osteoarthritis, hypertension, and altered kidney function.[17,25] In addition, although harder to measure, obesity exacerbates existing musculoskeletal problems, brachycephalic syndrome, and pregnancy, and is associated with increased anesthetic risk (Figure 1.2).

Fat as an Endocrine Organ

In addition to functioning as an energy storage site and thermal insulation, adipose tissue operates as an active endocrine organ. A variety of endocrine, paracrine, and autocrine signals are released from cells within adipose tissues. These signals are referred to as adipokines. The term adipokine is generally used to mean any protein released by adipose tissue regardless of whether it is released by adipocytes or non-fat cells.[26] To date, approximately 100 adipokines have been identified as being released from fat tissue, of which at least 24 have increased circulating levels in obese humans.[27,28] Some of these putative adipokines, such as C-reactive protein (CRP), haptoglobin, and amyloid A, are actually acute phase proteins primarily released by the liver in response to the mild inflammatory response seen in human obesity. Most of the remaining 21 also are inflammatory proteins, but the source of their elevated circulating levels in obesity is unclear and could result from release by tissues other than fat.[28]

Upregulation of the systemic inflammatory response appears to provide a critical pathophysiologic link to the wide variety of chronic diseases associated with obesity. There is increasing evidence that obesity in humans is associated with low-level inflammation that is often accompanied by hypertension and type-2 diabetes. Interestingly, some adipokines may actually have anti-inflammatory effects and circulate at higher levels in obesity as part of a homeostatic mechanism to counteract the effects of the inflammatory mediators. Interleukin 10 (IL-10) probably is such a molecule, and there is some evidence that interleukin 6 (IL-6) has dual effects.[28] Currently it is thought that the increase in visceral omental rather than abdominal subcutaneous adipose tissue best correlates with measures of insulin resistance and cardiovascular disease.[28] The state of low-grade systemic inflammation that accompanies obesity, as measured by assaying various adipokines, has now been shown in dogs to undergo reversal when weight loss occurs.[29]

Although many adipokines have been discovered, the function and physiologic relevance of most have not been identified. A handful of adipokines have been intensively studied and appear to positively or negatively impact insulin sensitivity. The metabolic role of most adipokines is complex and incompletely understood. The following are examples of adipokines that have been widely studied and have significant metabolic effects.

Leptin

The presence of an obesity mutation (ob) was first discovered in mice nearly 60 years ago.[30] Mice with the ob/ob mutation in the leptin gene are morbidly obese, insulin resistant, hypothyroid, infertile, and have defective T-cell immunity.[31] In 1994, this mutation was cloned, sequenced, and later found to code for the hormone leptin.[32] Leptin was the first adipokine identified, and its main function is to regulate body fat mass through appetite control and increased energy metabolism. As body fat mass increases, more leptin is secreted from adipocytes.[33] Leptin is able to cross the blood-brain barrier; it inhibits neurotransmitters that increase appetite and lower energy expenditure and stimulates neurons that decrease appetite and increase in energy expenditure.[34,35] Therefore, as individuals gain body fat, leptin promotes weight loss. Leptin has been called a "lipostat" because it works like a thermostat for body fat mass.[36,37] Although leptin's primary physiologic role is to regulate body fat storage, it also affects the immune, cardiovascular, and reproductive systems. In addition, leptin is capable of regulating cardiac and vascular contractility through a local nitric-oxide-dependent mechanism.[38,39]

Leptin also may enhance insulin signaling to improve intracellular glucose uptake and decrease the accumulation of lipid in peripheral tissues.[40] Lipid accumulation with cells can lead to the phenomenon of lipotoxicity, which has been implicated in the development of peripheral insulin resistance.[41,42] Administration of leptin decreases cellular lipid stores in the pancreas, adipose, liver, and cardiac tissues of rodents.[43] Leptin deficiencies found in *ob/ob* rodents result in obesity, insulin resistance, and diabetes.[44]

As evidenced by the current obesity epidemic, leptin does not always succeed in maintaining appropriate body fat mass. In fact, obese individuals often have the highest concentrations of this hormone.[45] When leptin cannot effectively regulate appetite and energy expenditure, this is termed "leptin resistance."[46] Several mechanisms may lead to leptin resistance: genetic mutation, receptor down-regulation, decreased permeation of the blood brain barrier, and molecular interference.[47] Although genetic mutations of leptin receptors can occur in humans, they are rare and account for only a tiny fraction of people with leptin resistance.

Leptin is capable of self-regulating its physiologic action by down-regulating its receptors. A reduction in receptor numbers has been demonstrated in the hypothalamus of rodents that overexpress leptin.[47] In addition, prolonged increases in central leptin concentrations eventually diminish its physiologic actions.[48] Evidence suggests that central leptin resistance causes obesity and that obesity-induced leptin resistance injures numerous peripheral tissues, including liver, pancreas, platelets, vasculature, and myocardium. This metabolic- and inflammatory-mediated injury may result from either resistance to leptin's action in selective tissues, or excess leptin action from adiposity-associated hyperleptinemia. In this sense, the term "leptin resistance" encompasses a complex pathophysiological phenomenon. The leptin axis has functional interactions with elements of metabolism, such as insulin, and inflammation, including mediators of innate immunity, such as interleukin-6. Plasma levels of leptin and inflammatory markers are correlated and also predict cardiovascular risk in human patients.[47]

Adiponectin

Adiponectin is the most abundantly secreted adipokine in circulation with concentrations in the µg/ml range (three orders of magnitude higher than leptin).[49] Although adipocytes are responsible for secreting adiponectin, hormone levels become paradoxically lower with increased fat mass.[50] The reason behind this unusual relationship is not clear. It is speculated that increased levels of other adipokines, such as tumor necrosis factor-alpha (TNF-α), may suppress adiponectin expression. Adiponectin exerts a myriad of metabolic affects. Perhaps the most influential role of adiponectin is as an insulin sensitizer. Adiponectin is closely associated with insulin sensitivity, independent of body fat mass.[51-53]

In a study of obese rhesus monkeys, low adiponectin levels correlated with insulin resistance and preceded the onset of diabetes mellitus.[54] Prospective and longitudinal studies in human beings also demonstrate that lower adiponectin levels are closely associated with insulin resistance and future development of diabetes.[55–57] Higher levels of adiponectin are also strongly associated with reduced risk of type-2 diabetes in healthy adult human beings.[58]

Adiponectin proteins bind to each other to form complexes of varying sizes. The high molecular weight (HMW) form of adiponectin is made up of 12 or more adiponectin molecules bound together. This HMW complex is thought to be the most active form of adiponectin and is more closely associated with insulin resistance and diabetes than total adiponectin or the lower weight forms.[59,60]

Numerous clinical and epidemiological studies associate low levels of adiponectin with chronic inflammatory states such as obesity, insulin-resistance, type-2 diabetes, hypertension, cardiovascular disease and liver disease.[61,62] Adiponectin is an attractive therapeutic target. In support of its therapeutic potential, administration of recombinant adiponectin ameliorates metabolic complications in mice, and the beneficial effects of the insulin-sensitizing thiazolodinedione drugs in human patients are at least partly due to the improvement in adiponectin profiles.[63]

Tumor Necrosis Factor-alpha

TNF-α is an inflammatory cytokine expressed by a variety of cells including macrophages, mast cells, neuronal cells, fibroblasts, and adipocytes. The connection between TNF-α, obesity, and insulin resistance is unclear. Because TNF-α can be secreted by both differentiated and undifferentiated adipocytes, it was thought that the increased levels of TNF-α found in obesity were primarily due to adipocyte secretion; however, cells within the stromovascular fraction of adipose tissue, including macrophages, produce significantly more TNF-α than adipocytes.[64–66] Obesity increases macrophage migration into adipose tissue, and this is likely the cause of increased TNF-α expression.[67,68] One theory behind recruitment of monocytes and macrophages to expanding adipose tissue is that increased levels of adipocyte apoptosis and necrosis produce chemoattractant agents.[65,69]

TNF-α secretion from adipose tissue has key species differences. In mice, TNF-α is released into systemic circulation.[69] In humans, most adipose TNF-α exerts local paracrine and autocrine actions.[70,71] Obese dogs tend to have higher systemic concentrations of TNF-α.[72] The circulation patterns of TNF-α derived from adipose tissue are not well understood in cats, but mRNA expression within fat is increased with obesity.[73]

One of the primary actions of adipose TNF-α is induction of localized insulin resistance. TNF-α down-regulates genes responsible for insulin-mediated glucose uptake into cells.[74–76] In addition to inhibiting glucose entry into cells, TNF-α decreases uptake of free fatty acids (FFA) into adipocytes and promotes lipolysis and release of FFA into circulation.[65,70,77] As a result, FFA levels increase in circulation and negatively affect insulin sensitivity in peripheral tissues.

In addition to directly influencing insulin sensitivity of adipose tissue, TNF-α can alter secretion of other adipokines involved in glucose metabolism. In particular, TNF-α inversely correlates with adiponectin and may alter its gene expression.[65,70,78,79] In contrast to adiponectin, expression of leptin and several other adipokines is increased by TNF-α.[80] In summary, TNF-α secreted from adipose tissue plays an important role in glucose and lipid metabolism at both the local and systemic levels and is a key component to inflammation associated with obesity.

Interleukin-6

Interleukin-6 (IL-6) is a pleiotropic cytokine affecting a wide variety of physiologic processes. It plays a major role in regulating inflammation, immune responses, and hematopoiesis.[81] IL-6 appears to mirror TNF-α in its interactions with other adipokines. It has an inhibitory effect on adiponectin and promotes expression of leptin, resistin, and visfatin.[80] Adipose tissue secretes up to 35% of basal IL-6 plasma levels.[71] Although adipocytes produce IL-6, other cells in the stromovascular fraction of adipose tissue also secrete the cytokine and probably contribute more to overall secretion.[81,82] Visceral adipose tissue secretes more IL-6 than subcutaneous adipose, and the concentration of IL-6 in adipose tissue is approximately 100-fold greater than that of plasma.[82,83] This implies that IL-6 plays an autocrine and/or paracrine role in adipose. One important function may be to induce lipolysis within adipocytes. Adipocytes and adipose tissue grown in culture with IL-6 demonstrate increased levels of lipolysis.[81,84] In addition, infusion of IL-6 in humans increases overall fatty acid concentration and oxidation.[81,85,86]

Several studies[87–89] demonstrate a positive relationship between IL-6 adipose expression and insulin resistance; however, a cause-and-effect relationship has not been established, and higher concentrations of IL-6 may only reflect increased adipocyte numbers. Studies showing that IL-6 closely correlates with body mass index (BMI) but not insulin sensitivity in healthy and diabetic patients support this idea.[90,91] Some of the confusion regarding IL-6's contribution to insulin sensitivity may be due to its conflicting action on the skeletal muscle, liver, and fat. In general, IL-6 appears to improve insulin's action in skeletal muscle while impairing insulin-mediated glycogen synthesis and glucose uptake in hepatic and adipose tissue, respectively.[81]

Appetite Regulation

Obesity occurs when more calories are consumed than the body needs. Understanding factors that influence the amount of food eaten is key to preventing and managing obesity. The three main components that determine food intake are environment, emotional or cognitive decisions, and metabolic regulation. Pet owners have the most control over the environment by limiting the amount of food available to their pets. However, owner compliance improves when we consider the emotional and metabolic aspects of food intake. For example, part of the reason dogs enjoy receiving treats from their caregivers is the extra attention that is given. The joy of getting a treat may be replaced with owner praise and affection in many instances. The emotional role of food intake has been studied extensively in humans and is influenced by many factors including depression, boredom, palatability, serving dish size, and social situations.[92,93]

Although it is difficult to assess many of the thoughts and emotions dogs and cats undergo while eating, some of the same factors probably influence their food intake. Cats living in apartments are more likely to be obese, and although activity level certainly impacts their weight, boredom or lack of environmental enrichment also may lead to increased food intake.[16] Increased exercise and activity may fight obesity in pets by burning extra calories and improving the emotional health of cats and dogs. The metabolic controls of appetite and food intake are numerous and complex. This discussion focuses only on a few key aspects.

The arcuate nucleus of the hypothalamus is the main central regulator of appetite. Within the arcuate nucleus there are two sets of neurons that have opposing actions. Anorexigenic neurons inhibit appetite and include the proopiomelanocortin (POMC) and cocaine-amphetamine regulated transcript (CART) neurons. The anorexigenic neurons release α-MSH, which decreases food intake and increases energy expenditure by acting on melanocortin receptors (MC3 and MC4). Orexigenic neurons increase food intake and include neuropeptide Y (NPY) and agouti-related gene transcript (AgRP). NPY inhibits POMC cells. AgRP antagonizes MC3 and MC4 receptors and reduces the anorectic effects of α-melanocyte stimulating hormone (α-MSH) (Figure 1.3). The appetite-regulating neurons in the hypothalamus are influenced by peripheral signals such as leptin and by other centers in the brain.[94]

Peripheral controls of appetite involve the entire body. The mouth is the first contact food has with the body, and when food touches the tongue or palate it stimulates the brain to continue or stop eating. Oral stimulation of acceptable food encourages food intake through cranial nerve and olfactory sensors. Dopamine and opiods are the main neurotransmitters mediating positive feedback of oral stimuli. As food moves into the stomach, a hormone called ghrelin is secreted from the gastric mucosa. Levels of ghrelin peak just before a meal is eaten and

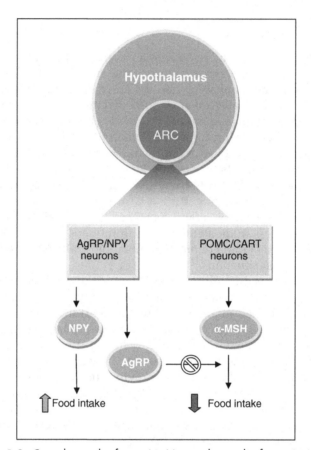

Figure 1.3. Central controls of appetite. Neuronal controls of appetite in the arcuate nucleus (ARC) within the hypothalamus of the brain. Neuropeptide Y (NPY) and agouti-related protein (AgRP) are released from neurons that stimulate appetite. Proopiomelanocortin (POMC) and cocaine-amphetamine regulated transcript (CART) neurons release α-melanocyte stimulating hormone (α-MSH), which suppresses appetite. AgRP inhibits the action of α-MSH.

rapidly decrease as nutrients enter the duodenum. It directly affects the reward system in the brain and is responsible for initiating hunger and food-seeking behaviors. While ghrelin stimulates appetite, most other signals from the gastrointestinal tract suppress feeding behavior. As the stomach expands with food, mechanoreceptors of the vagus nerve and spinal visceral afferent fibers are activated and cause release of anorexigenic peptides.[95] This is the mechanism behind the satiating effects of foods high in fiber and moisture that tend to fill the stomach without providing nutrient energy.

As nutrients move into the small intestine, proteins, monosaccharides, and fatty acids act on mucosal receptors that stimulate vagal afferent nerves and endocrine cells. Some of the key hormones released from the small intestine are cholecystokinin (CCK), glucagon-like peptide 1 (GLP-1), and protein YY (PYY). CCK release is stimulated mostly by fats and proteins and it works by slowing gastrointestinal motility and gastric emptying. It also stimulates the vagus nerve to suppress appetite. PYY is found throughout the human intestinal tract and increases distally. The colon and rectum have the highest concentrations. PYY is released after meals from L cells in the intestine and its concentrations peak two hours after a meal. Therefore, PYY may be important in regulating the timing of meals. GLP-1 is released into circulation after a meal and is co-secreted from L cells with PYY. GLP-1 is an incretin (promotes insulin release) and also acts on the hypothalamus and the brain stem-vagus system. The pancreas also impacts appetite with its release of insulin and amylin during and after meals.[95] Insulin and amylin decrease eating through central actions that result from their cumulative release over time. As mentioned earlier, adipose tissue also regulates appetite through the release of the hormone leptin. As adipose tissue increases, leptin is released and suppresses appetite.[96]

In Practice

Explaining the health risks associated with obesity will help clients understand the importance of helping their pet's return to or maintenance of an ideal body weight.

- Obesity is a pro-inflammatory state due to cytokines released from fat. Hormones produced by fat contribute to the detrimental health effects of obesity.
- Excess body weight shortens life span. In dogs, this has been shown to be about a 15% reduction.
- Obesity has known health risks for some serious diseases that can influence both quality of life and life span in pets. Significant illnesses associated with obesity/overweight in dogs are cranial cruciate injury, osteoarthritis, and pancreatitis; in cats, these are diabetes mellitus, lower urinary tract disorders, and hepatic lipidosis.
- Diets with low caloric density that are high in fiber and moisture may help suppress appetite by stimulating stomach mechanoreceptors. Diets containing fats and proteins can decrease appetite through the release of CCK.

References

1. Stanton C, Hamar D, Johnson D, et al. 1992. Bioelectrical impedance and zoometry for body composition analysis in domestic cats. *Am J Vet Res* 53:251–256.

2. Laflamme DP, Kuhlman G, Lawler DF, et al. 1994. Obesity management in dogs. *Veterinary Clinical Nutrition* 1:59,62–65.

3. Laflamme DP, Kuhlman G, Lawler DF. 1997. Evaluation of weight loss protocols for dogs. *Journal of the American Animal Hospital Association* 33:253–259.

4. Laflamme D. 1997. Development and validation of a body condition score system for cats: A clinical tool. *Feline Practice* 25:13–18.

5. Laflamme D. 1997. Nutritional management. *Veterinary Clinics of North America, Small Animal Practice* 27:1561–1577.

6. Toll P, Yamka R, Schoenherr W, et al. 2010. Obesity. In: Hand M, Thatcher C, Remillard R, et al., eds. *Small Animal Clinical Nutrition*, V ed. Topeka, KS: Mark Morris Institute, 501–544.

7. Toll P, Burkholder W. 2000. Obesity. In: Hand M, Thatcher C, Remillard R, et al., eds. *Small Animal Clinical Nutrition*, IV ed. Topeka, KS: Mark Morris Institute, 401–430.

8. Butterwick R. 2000. How fat is that cat? *J Feline Med Surg* 2:91–94.

9. Laflamme D. 1997. Development and validation of a body condition score system for dogs. *Canine Practice* 22:10–15.

10. German AJ, Holden SL, Moxham GL, et al. 2006. A simple, reliable tool for owners to assess the body condition of their dog or cat. *Journal of Nutrition* 136:2031S-2033S.

11. Thatcher C, Hand M, Remillard R. 2010. Small Animal Clinical Nutrition: An Iterative Process. In: Hand M, Thatcher C, Remillard R, et al., eds. *Small Animal Clinical Nutrition*, V ed. Topeka, KS: Mark Morris Institute, 3–21.

12. Lusby A, Kirk C. Obesity. 2008. *Kirk's Current Veterinary Therapy, XIV*: St. Louis: Saunders Elsevier, 191–196.

13. Michel KE, Sorenmo K, Shofer FS. 2004. Evaluation of body condition and weight loss in dogs presented to a veterinary oncology service. *Journal of Veterinary Internal Medicine* 18:692–695.

14. Baez JL, Michel KE, Sorenmo K, et al. 2007. A prospective investigation of the prevalence and prognostic significance of weight loss and changes in body condition in feline cancer patients. *Journal of Feline Medicine and Surgery* 9:411–417.

15. McGreevy PD, Thomson PC, Pride C, et al. 2005. Prevalence of obesity in dogs examined by Australian veterinary practices and the risk factors involved. *Veterinary Record* 156:695–702.

16. Lund E, Armstrong P, Kirk C, et al. 2005. Prevalence and risk factors for obesity in adult cats from private US veterinary practices. *Intern J Appl Res Vet Med* 3:88–96.

17. Lund EM, Armstrong PJ, Kirk CA, et al. 2006. Prevalence and risk factors for obesity in adult dogs from private US veterinary practices. *International Journal of Applied Research in Veterinary Medicine* 4:177–186.

18. Root MV, Johnston SD, Olson PN. 1996. Effect of prepuberal and postpuberal gonadectomy on heat production measured by indirect calorimetry in male and female domestic cats. *American Journal of Veterinary Research* 57:371–374.

19. ten Hacken NHT. 2009. Physical inactivity and obesity: Relation to asthma and chronic obstructive pulmonary disease? *Proc Am Thorac Soc* 6:663–667.

20. Fulop T, Tessier D, Carpentier A. 2006. The metabolic syndrome. *Pathologie Biologie* 54:375–386.

21. Teucher B, Rohrmann S, Kaaks R. 2010. Obesity: Focus on all-cause mortality and cancer. *Maturitas* 65:112–116.

22. Guh D, Zhang W, Bansback N, et al. 2009. The incidence of co-morbidities related to obesity and overweight: A systematic review and meta-analysis. *BMC Public Health* 9:88.

23. Kealy RD, Lawler DF, Ballam JM, et al. 2002. Effects of diet restriction on life span and age-related changes in dogs. *Journal of the American Veterinary Medical Association* 220:1315–1320.

24. Scarlett J, Donoghue S. 1998. Associations between body condition and disease in cats. *J Am Vet Med Assoc* 212:1725–1731.

25. Perez Alenza MD, Pena L, Castillo ND, et al. 2000. Factors influencing the incidence and prognosis of canine mammary tumours. *Journal of Small Animal Practice* 41:287–291.

26. Fain JN, Tagele BM, Cheema P, et al. 2010. Release of 12 adipokines by adipose tissue, nonfat cells, and fat cells from obese women. *Obesity* 18:890–896.

27. Halberg N, Wernstedt-Asterholm I, Scherer PE. 2008. The adipocyte as an endocrine cell. *Endocrinology and Metabolism Clinics of North America* 37:753–768.

28. Fain JN. 2010. Release of inflammatory mediators by human adipose tissue is enhanced in obesity and primarily by the nonfat cells: A review. *Mediators Inflamm* 2010.

29. Yamka R, Friesen K, Frantz N. 2006. Identification of canine markers related to obesity and the effects of weight loss on the markers of interest. *Intern J Appl Res Vet Med* 4:282–292.

30. Ingalls AM, Dickie MM, Snell GD. 1950. Obese, a new mutation in the house mouse. *J Hered* 41:317–318.

31. Oswal A, Yeo GSH. 2007. The leptin melanocortin pathway and the control of body weight: Lessons from human and murine genetics. *Obes Rev* 8:293–306.

32. Zhang Y, Proenca R, Maffei M, et al. 1994. Positional cloning of the mouse obese gene and its human homologue. *Nature* 372:425–432.

33. Zhang F, Chen Y, Heiman M, et al. 2005. Leptin: Structure, Function and Biology. *Vitamins and Hormones*. London: Academic Press, 345–372.

34. Oswal A, Yeo GSH. 2007. The leptin melanocortin pathway and the control of body weight: Lessons from human and murine genetics. *Obesity Reviews* 8:293–306.

35. Horvath TL. 2006. Synaptic plasticity in energy balance regulation. *Obesity* 14:228S-233.

36. Lusby AL, Kirk CA, Bartges JW. 2009. The role of key adipokines in obesity and insulin resistance in cats. *Journal of the American Veterinary Medical Association* 235:518–522.

37. Anukulkitch C, Rao A, Dunshea F, et al. 2009. A test of the lipostat theory in a seasonal (ovine) model under natural conditions reveals a close relationship between adiposity and melanin concentrating hormone expression. *Domest Anim Endocrinol* 36:138–151.

38. Ren J. 2004. Leptin and hyperleptinemia—from friend to foe for cardiovascular function. *J Endocrinol* 181:1–10.

39. Munzberg H, Myers Jr. MG. 2005. Molecular and anatomical determinants of central leptin resistance. *Nat Neurosci* 8:566–570.

40. Park S, Hong SM, Sung SR, et al. 2007. Long-term effects of central leptin and resistin on body weight, insulin resistance, and {beta}-cell function and mass by the modulation of hypothalamic leptin and insulin signaling. *Endocrinology* 2007-0754.

41. Griffin ME, Marcucci MJ, Cline GW, et al. 1999. Free fatty acid-induced insulin resistance is associated with activation of protein kinase C theta and alterations in the insulin signaling cascade. *Diabetes* 48:1270–1274.

42. Boden G. 2003. Effects of free fatty acids (FFA) on glucose metabolism: significance for insulin resistance and type 2 diabetes. *Experimental and Clinical Endocrinology & Diabetes* 111:121–124.

43. Dyck DJ, Heigenhauser GJF, Bruce CR. 2006. The role of adipokines as regulators of skeletal muscle fatty acid metabolism and insulin sensitivity. *Acta Physiologica* 186:5–16.

44. Sell H, Dietze-Schroeder D, Eckel J. 2006. The adipocyte-myocyte axis in insulin resistance. *Trends Endocrinol Metab* 17:416–422.

45. Münzberg H, Björnholm M, Bates SH, et al. 2005. Leptin receptor action and mechanisms of leptin resistance. *Cellular and Molecular Life Sciences (CMLS)* 62:642–652.

46. Shimizu H, Oh-I S, Okada S, et al. 2007. Leptin resistance and obesity. *Endocrine J* 54:17–26.

47. Martin SS, Qasim A, Reilly MP. 2008. Leptin resistance: A possible interface of inflammation and metabolism in obesity-related cardiovascular disease. *J Am Colleg Cardiol* 52:1201–1210.

48. Scarpace PJ, Matheny M, Tümer N, et al. 2005. Leptin resistance exacerbates diet-induced obesity and is associated with diminished maximal leptin signalling capacity in rats. *Diabetologia* 48:1075–1083.

49. Whitehead JP, Richards AA, Hickman IJ, et al. 2006. Adiponectin—a key adipokine in the metabolic syndrome. *Diabetes Obes Metab* 8:264–280.

50. Arita Y, Kihara S, Ouchi N, et al. 1999. Paradoxical decrease of an adipose-specific protein, adiponectin, in obesity. *Biochem Biophysical Res Comm* 257:79–83.

51. Weyer C, Funahashi T, Tanaka S, et al. 2001. Hypoadiponectinemia in obesity and type 2 diabetes: Close association with insulin resistance and hyperinsulinemia. *J Clin Endocrinol Metab* 86:1930–1935.

52. Kantartzis K, Fritsche A, Tschritter O, et al. 2005. The association between plasma adiponectin and insulin sensitivity in humans depends on obesity. *Obesity Res* 13:1683–1691.

53. Tschritter O, Fritsche A, Thamer C, et al. 2003. Plasma adiponectin concentrations predict insulin sensitivity of both glucose and lipid metabolism. *Diabetes* 52:239–243.
54. Hotta K, Funahashi T, Bodkin NL, et al. 2001. Circulating concentrations of the adipocyte protein adiponectin are decreased in parallel with reduced insulin sensitivity during the progression to type 2 diabetes in rhesus monkeys. *Diabetes* 50:1126–1133.
55. Lindsay RS, Funahashi T, Hanson RL, et al. 2002. Adiponectin and development of type 2 diabetes in the Pima Indian population. *Lancet* 360:57–58.
56. Yamamoto Y, Hirose H, Saito I, et al. 2004. Adiponectin, an adipocyte-derived protein, predicts future insulin resistance: Two-year follow-up study in Japanese population. *J Clin Endocrinol Metab* 89:87–90.
57. Snehalatha C, Mukesh B, Simon M, et al. 2003. Plasma adiponectin is an independent predictor of type 2 diabetes in Asian Indians. *Diabetes Care* 26:3226–3229.
58. Spranger J, Kroke A, Mohlig M, et al. 2003. Adiponectin and protection against type 2 diabetes mellitus. *Lancet* 361:226–228.
59. Pajvani UB, Hawkins M, Combs TP, et al. 2004. Complex distribution, not absolute amount of adiponectin, correlates with thiazolidinedione-mediated improvement in insulin sensitivity. *J Biol Chem* 279:12152–12162.
60. Fisher M, Trujillo M, Hanif W, et al. 2005. Serum high molecular weight complex of adiponectin correlates better with glucose tolerance than total serum adiponectin in Indo-Asian males. *Diabetologia* 48:1084–1087.
61. Greenberg AS, Obin MS. 2006. Obesity and the role of adipose tissue in inflammation and metabolism. *Am J Clin Nutr* 83:461S-465.
62. Ouchi N, Walsh K. 2007. Adiponectin as an anti-inflammatory factor. *Clinica Chimica Acta* 380:24–30.
63. Phillips SA, Kung JT. 2010. Mechanisms of adiponectin regulation and use as a pharmacological target. *Current Opinion in Pharmacology* 10:676–683.
64. Weisberg SP, McCann D, Desai M, Rosenbaum M, Leibel RL, Ferrante AW. 2003. Obesity is associated with macrophage accumulation in adipose tissue. *J Clin Invest* 112:1796–1808.
65. Cawthorn WP, Sethi JK. 2008. TNF-[alpha] and adipocyte biology. *FEBS Letters* 582:117–131.
66. Fain JN, Bahouth SW, Madan AK. 2004. TNF[alpha] release by the nonfat cells of human adipose tissue. *Int J Obes Relat Metab Disord* 28:616–622.
67. Coenen KR, Gruen ML, Chait A, et al. 2007. Diet-induced increases in adiposity, but not plasma lipids, promote macrophage infiltration into white adipose tissue. *Diabetes* 56:564–573.
68. Weisberg SP, McCann D, Desai M, et al. 2003. Obesity is associated with macrophage accumulation in adipose tissue. *J Clin Invest* 112:1796–1808.
69. Hotamisligil GS, Shargill NS, Spiegelman BM. 1993. Adipose expression of tumor necrosis factor-alpha: direct role in obesity-linked insulin resistance. *Science* 259:87–91.

70. Ryden M, Arner P. 2007. Tumour necrosis factor-alpha in human adipose tissue—from signalling mechanisms to clinical implications. *J Internal Med* 262:431–438.

71. Mohamed-Ali V, Goodrick S, Rawesh A, et al. 1997. Subcutaneous adipose tissue releases interleukin-6, but not tumor necrosis factor-{alpha}, *in vivo*. *J Clin Endocrinol Metab* 82:4196–4200.

72. German AJ, Hervera M, Hunter L, et al. 2009. Improvement in insulin resistance and reduction in plasma inflammatory adipokines after weight loss in obese dogs. *Domestic Animal Endocrinology* 37:214–226.

73. Hoenig M, McGoldrick JB, deBeer M, et al. 2006. Activity and tissue-specific expression of lipases and tumor-necrosis factor [alpha] in lean and obese cats. *Dom Anim Endocrinol* 30:333–344.

74. Stephens JM, Lee J, Pilch PF. 1997. Tumor necrosis factor-alpha-induced insulin resistance in 3T3-L1 adipocytes is accompanied by a loss of insulin receptor substrate-1 and GLUT4 expression without a loss of insulin receptor-mediated signal transduction. *J Biol Chem* 272:971–976.

75. Qi C, Pekala PH. 2000. Tumor necrosis factor-alpha induced insulin resistance in adipocytes. *Proc Soc Exp Biol Med* 223:128–135.

76. Peraldi P, Xu M, Spiegelman BM. 1997. Thiazolidinediones block tumor necrosis factor-alpha induced inhibition of insulin signaling. *J Clin Invest* 100:1863–1869.

77. Memon RA, Feingold KR, Moser AH, et al. 1998. Regulation of fatty acid transport protein and fatty acid translocase mRNA levels by endotoxin and cytokines. *Am J Physiol* 274:E210–E217.

78. Kita A, Yamasaki H, Kuwahara H, et al. 2005. Identification of the promoter region required for human adiponectin gene transcription: Association with CCAAT/enhancer binding protein-[beta] and tumor necrosis factor-[alpha]. *Biochem Biophys Res Commun* 331:484–490.

79. Kim K-Y, Kim JK, Jeon JH, et al. 2005. c-Jun N-terminal kinase is involved in the suppression of adiponectin expression by TNF-[alpha] in 3T3-L1 adipocytes. *Biochem Biophys Res Commun* 327:460–467.

80. Rabe K, Lehrke M, Parhofer K, et al. 2008. Adipokines and insulin resistance. *Mol Med* 14:741–751.

81. Hoene M, Weigert C. 2008. The role of interleukin-6 in insulin resistance, body fat distribution and energy balance. *Obesity Reviews* 9:20–2.

82. Fain JN, Madan AK, Hiler ML, et al. 2004. Comparison of the release of adipokines by adipose tissue, adipose tissue matrix, and adipocytes from visceral and subcutaneous abdominal adipose tissues of obese humans. *Endocrinol* 145:2273–2282.

83. Sopasakis VR, Sandqvist M, Gustafson B, et al. 2004. High local concentrations and effects on differentiation implicate interleukin-6 as a paracrine regulator. *Obesity Res* 12:454–460.

84. Trujillo ME, Sullivan S, Harten I, et al. 2004. Interleukin-6 regulates human adipose tissue lipid metabolism and leptin production *in vitro*. *J Clin Endocrinol Metab* 89:5577–5582.

85. Lyngso D, Simonsen L, Bulow J. 2002. Metabolic effects of interleukin-6 in human splanchnic and adipose tissue. *J Physiol* 543:379–386.
86. Van Hall G, Steensberg A, Sacchetti M, et al. 2003. Interleukin-6 stimulates lipolysis and fat oxidation in humans. *J Clin Endocrinol Metab* 88:3005–3010.
87. Kern PA, Ranganathan S, Li C, et al. 2001. Adipose tissue tumor necrosis factor and interleukin-6 expression in human obesity and insulin resistance. *Am J Physiol Endocrinol Metab* 280:E745–751.
88. Rotter V, Nagaev I, Smith U. 2003. Interleukin-6 (IL-6) induces insulin resistance in 3T3-L1 adipocytes and is, like IL-8 and tumor necrosis factor-{alpha}, overexpressed in human fat cells from insulin-resistant subjects. *J Biol Chem* 278:45777–45784.
89. Carey AL, Febbraio MA. 2004. Interleukin-6 and insulin sensitivity: Friend or foe? *Diabetologia* 47:1135–1142.
90. Carey AL, Bruce CR, Sacchetti M, et al. 2004. Interleukin-6 and tumor necrosis factor-a are not increased in patients with Type 2 diabetes: Evidence that plasma interleukin-6 is related to fat mass and not insulin responsiveness. *Diabetologia* 47:1029–1037.
91. Vozarova B, Weyer C, Hanson K, et al. 2001. Circulating interleukin-6 in relation to adiposity, insulin action, and insulin secretion. *Obesity Res* 9:414–417.
92. Konttinen H, Silventoinen K, Sarlio-Lahteenkorva S, et al. 2010. Emotional eating and physical activity self-efficacy as pathways in the association between depressive symptoms and adiposity indicators. *Am J Clin Nutr* 92:1031–1039.
93. Wansink B. 2010. From mindless eating to mindlessly eating better. *Physiology and Behavior* 100:454–463.
94. Suzuki K, Simpson KA, Minnion JS, et al. 2010. The role of gut hormones and the hypothalamus in appetite regulation. *Endocrine Journal* 57:359–372.
95. Chaudhri OB, Field BCT, Bloom SR. 2008. Gastrointestinal satiety signals. *International Journal of Obesity* 32:S28-S31.
96. Kalra SP, Kalra PS. 2010. Neuroendocrine Control of Energy Homeostasis: Update on New Insights. In: Luciano M, ed. *Progress in Brain Research*: Oxford, UK: Elsevier, 17–33.

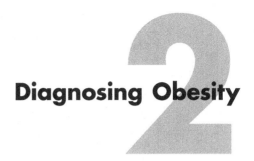

Diagnosing Obesity

Todd L. Towell, DVM, MS, DACVIM

Recognizing a Problem: The First Step to Solving It

It has been said that pets, particularly dogs, look like their owners. Sadly, in recent years, this has come to mean that most are overweight and suffering numerous health consequences just like us. In the United States roughly 30% of adults and 20% of children are obese.[1,2] One contributing factor to the rise of obesity in humans may be lack of recognition both by patients and physicians.

Although adults are relatively accurate in assessing their own body condition, parents of overweight children invariably underestimate their children's weight. Even when mothers correctly identify themselves as overweight they fail to correctly identify their child's weight status as overweight or obese.[3] This phenomenon has been documented in more than 15 recent studies.[3,4] In one study only 10.5% of parents of overweight children perceived their child's weight accurately. Recognition of a problem is the first step to solving it. Given that most parents of overweight children fail to recognize their child has a weight problem, it is incumbent upon the medical profession to diagnose and recommended treatment for these individuals.

In people, body mass index (BMI) is a useful tool for diagnosing and classifying the degree of overweight and obesity. BMI describes relative weight for height and is calculated by dividing body weight (kg) by height squared (m^2). The resultant BMI value is not the same as percent body fat but is significantly correlated with body fat content (Table 2.1). Patients with BMI 25 to 29.9 are considered overweight and patients

Table 2.1. Human overweight and obesity classifications.

Class	Obese class	BMI (kg/m2)
Underweight	–	<18.5
Normal	–	18.5–24.9
Overweight	–	25–29.9
Obesity	I	30–34.9
	II	35–39.9
Extreme obesity	III	≥40

with BMI greater than 30 are considered obese. In children, overweight is defined as a BMI between the 85th and 95th percentile, and obesity is defined as a BMI in the 95th percentile or higher for children of the same age and sex. These distinctions are important because early intervention is associated with decreased risk of complications. Ideally, all patients with BMI greater than 25 for adults or children in or above the 85th percentile would receive recommendations for weight loss.

However, in a recent study of patient visits to private physician offices and hospital outpatient departments, only 29% of adults who were obese according to their BMI had a documented diagnosis of obesity.[5] The proportion of patients with a diagnosis of obesity increased with increasing BMI from 19% for patients between 30 and 34.9 to 50% for those whose BMI was 40 or greater. A similar study designed to assess how often general pediatricians, pediatric endocrinologists, and gastroenterologists diagnose children as overweight found only 31% of obese children were diagnosed as such.[6] Most discouragingly, the patients most likely to benefit from early interventions, children with a BMI percentile of 85% to 94%, were also those least likely to receive a diagnosis and recommendations for intervention.[6] These results indicate that in human medicine obesity is underappreciated in clinical practice. Physicians both fail to obtain needed patient data and fail to clinically identify obesity even when data that are obtained suggest this disease is present.

The situation is not much better for pets. Estimates have suggested that between 34% and 52% of the dogs and cats are overweight or obese.[7-9] Based on the results of a 2008 survey of 95 veterinary clinics, The Association for Pet Obesity Prevention (APOP) estimates that in the U.S., more than 44% of dogs and 57% of cats are now overweight or obese (Figure 2.1). According to this study, this translates into 7.2 million obese and 26 million overweight dogs. The number in cats is even higher, with 15.7 million obese and 35 million overweight cats. Veterinarians routinely rise to the challenge of diagnosing diseases with subtle clinical signs in nonverbal patients. However, just like our physician counterparts, many veterinarians fail to diagnose one of the most easily recognizable diseases, obesity.

Key Point

Many veterinarians fail to diagnose one of the most easily recognizable diseases, obesity.

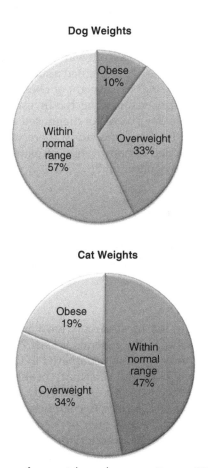

Dog Weights

Obese 10%

Within normal range 57%

Overweight 33%

Cat Weights

Obese 19%

Within normal range 47%

Overweight 34%

Figure 2.1. Percentage of overweight or obese pets. Source: 2007 Association for Pet Obesity Prevention Study.

How would you react if you knew that owners of pets in your practice were not being informed of abnormal results of routine blood chemistry and urinalysis? Is it ever appropriate to avoid discussing abnormal laboratory findings simply because the owner may not want to hear the results? If routine screening detected azotemia and inappropriately concentrated urine consistent with chronic kidney disease would you wait until next year's visit to see if the condition worsens before discussing findings with the owner? As absurd as these suggestions sound, this happens routinely with regard to abnormal body condition.

In one study veterinarians diagnosed 2% of dogs and 1.8% of cats as obese despite the fact that 28.3% of dogs and 27.5% of cats were assigned a body condition score that corresponded with overweight or obese.[10] A study designed to determine whether practitioners commonly assess body weight and body condition of dogs in their care found that while 70% of dogs were weighed, subjective body conditions were assessed in 29% and a body condition score was assigned only once during 2,000 consultations.[11] Of those dogs assigned a subjective body condition, 15% (22/148) were classified as overweight or obese, a much smaller proportion than recent estimates, leading the investigators to suggest many overweight or obese dogs were not diagnosed as such by their primary care veterinarian. In this same study there was a strong association between the frequency of bodyweight measurements and discussions about the dog's body condition.[11]

Key Point

It is a common misconception that the maximum BCS corresponds to a maximum amount of body fat.

Not surprisingly, like most parents, most owners underestimate their pet's body condition.[12-15] In general, at least 70% of owners underestimate their pet's body condition compared to the assessment of trained observers. In many cases the veterinary health care team may need to change an owners' perception of the body condition of their pet if weight loss is to be successful.[12] Two studies document that owners are more likely to correctly assess their pet's condition when using a visual scale compared to verbal descriptions.[14,15] Owners, like parents, are reluctant to use verbal descriptions that include terms with negative connotations (overweight and obese) to describe their pets. Perhaps of even more concern than the lack of awareness is the apparent lack of concern. A study designed to estimate disease prevalence among dogs and cats in the United States and Australia found that although 32% of owners self reported their pets were slightly overweight or obese, less than 1% (3/356) of these owners considered this to be a health problem.[16] Additionally, only nine of these pets (2.5%) were being fed a reduced-calorie or reduced-fat food.

Obviously, barriers to obesity screening and diagnosis exist for health care providers, both veterinarians and physicians. Despite recent studies and public health campaigns, some health care providers (veterinarians and physicians) and many patients/clients still may not consider an abnormal body condition a significant health concern. It is most likely that the diagnosis of abnormal body condition is overlooked because of a combination of health care provider and patient/client factors including lack of time for preventative care, lack of provider skills, lack of resources to address obesity, and provider/patient/client concerns about weight stigma.[5] Both physicians and veterinarians may fail to counsel patients/clients on obesity because of their frustration with weight loss programs they have recommended in the past.

Obesity is a complex chronic condition and the entire health care team plays an important role in preventing, identifying, and managing it. When veterinarians and veterinary health care team members truly believe that maintaining/achieving an ideal body weight will improve patients' quality of life and life expectancy, they will be more enthusiastic about discussing the topic with clients. Similarly, when clients understand the importance of maintaining an ideal weight to their pet's overall health, they will be more receptive to recommendations from the health care team.

Defining Obesity

Deciding that a cat or dog is overweight is usually not difficult; however, accurately determining the degree to which they are overweight and the patient's ideal weight can be challenging. The subjectivity associated with most clinical methods of assessing body fat makes accurate objective measurement problematic. Variations in body conformation across breeds, variations in frame size within breeds, and the veterinarian's and owner's bias for what constitutes ideal body weight all contribute to the problem.

By definition, obesity is the accumulation of excess body fat. Although body weight can increase for a variety of reasons, the majority of overweight dogs and cats are heavy because of excess body fat. People are considered obese when percent body fat (% BF) exceeds 20% to 30% of total weight.[17] Clinically in people, BMI is calculated from height and weight and used to estimate % BF. This mathematical estimation of % BF works reasonably well for people because as a species we have relatively similar body conformations, and extensive data on optimal height–weight standards exist for men and women. Not so in veterinary medicine. The ratio between the heaviest and lightest of well known cat breeds is 1:4, which is relatively homogenous compared to dogs, in which the ratio is 1:100 (Figure 2.2). This variation of frame size across and within breeds combined with the lack of data on optimal standards make determining % BF more challenging in veterinary patients.

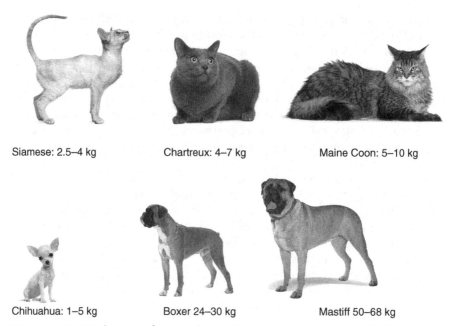

Siamese: 2.5–4 kg   Chartreux: 4–7 kg   Maine Coon: 5–10 kg

Chihuahua: 1–5 kg   Boxer 24–30 kg   Mastiff 50–68 kg

Figure 2.2. Weight ranges for several cat and dog breeds. Images from Fotolia.com.

Clinical Tools

Unfortunately, there is no single best method readily available in clinical practice for deciding if a pet has a thin, ideal, overweight, or obese body condition. The paradox is that having an objective assessment of body condition is vital for diagnosing obesity. In the absence of an objective method of diagnosis, convincing owners that their pet has a serious medical condition and will benefit from weight loss is nearly impossible. Visual cues such as radiographic or ultrasound images can illustrate the problem for owners but will not objectively quantify the degree to with the pet is overweight. All pets fall along a spectrum from emaciation to morbid obesity. Assigning absolute divisions is difficult and subjective.

Determining the extent of excess body weight and the pet's ideal body weight is the first essential step in an effective weight loss program. A variety of methods of assessing body condition are available (Table 2.2). Some are more clinically applicable than others. The following is a discussion of tools which can be easily used in clinical practice.

Relative Body Weight

One common way to determine obesity in veterinary patients is relative body weight (RBW), which is simply an animal's current weight divided by its estimated optimal weight. People are defined as mildly obese

Table 2.2. Methods used to estimate/determine body condition.

Clinical techniques	Research techniques	Techniques with limited clinical availability
Relative body weight	Chemical analysis	Dual energy X-ray absorptiometry
Body condition scoring	Dilution techniques	Computed tomography
Morphometric measurements	Total body potassium	Magnetic resonance imaging
Sequential body weight measurements/ photography	Densitometry	
Bioelectrical impedance analysis	Neutron activation analysis	

when actual body weight exceeds optimal body weight by 15% to 30%.[17] Similar ranges for relative body weight in dogs and cats have been determined. Dogs and cats with RBW 10% to 20% over optimal weight are considered overweight; those greater than 20% are considered obese. This technique is hampered by the fact that determining a pet's optimal weight is often challenging.

Body Condition Scoring

Body condition scoring (BCS) is perhaps the most commonly used system to estimate body fat in clinical practice. BCS is a subjective and semiquantitative method that combines visual assessment (from the top and side) and palpation (waist, ribs, and abdominal tuck, and dorsal spinous processes at tail base) to estimate adipose tissue mass. Body condition scoring systems take into account the pet's frame size independent of its weight. Although there are a number of validated scoring systems that use defined criteria to help objectify the process, this remains a subjective technique.

Like other physical examination techniques this is a learned skill. The scorer must learn through experience what visible and palpable cues correspond to a given BCS. For that reason consistency of scores between observers can be challenging. What one scorer feels to be an excessive amount of fat covering the ribs, another scorer may assess as appropriate. However, despite the subjective nature of assigning a BCS, once learned, it is a relatively reliable method for determining the proportion of body fat or body composition.[18] The advantage of BCS systems is they can be easily applied in the clinical setting and they aid both in the diagnosis and prevention of obesity.

Body condition scoring systems for dogs and cats using three to nine categories have been assessed for precision and accuracy.[19–23] Systems with either five or nine categories are most commonly used. A

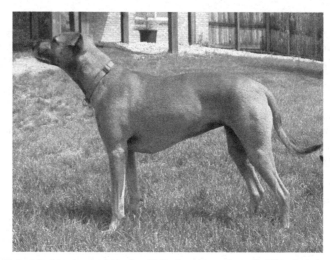

Figure 2.3. Ideal body condition for 40-lb dog. Note the well defined abdominal tuck and waist. Photo courtesy of Todd Towell.

nine-point system scored to the nearest whole score and a five-point system scored to the nearest half score both have nine total scores. In general, dogs and cats with ideal body condition should have:

1. Normal body contours and silhouettes (Figure 2.3)
2. Bony prominences that can be readily palpated but not seen or felt above skin surfaces
3. Intraabdominal fat insufficient to interfere with abdominal palpation

When the five-point system is scored to the nearest half score, it subdivides body condition into three broad categories: insufficient, ideal, and excess, with a score of 3 falling in the middle of the optimal range (Figure 2.4). The most critical division points in a five-point system are between the scores of 2 vs. 2.5 and 3.5 vs. 4 because assignment of a BCS less than 2.5 or greater than 3.5 suggests action should be taken to return the patient's BCS to the optimal range. These same criteria (i.e., what contours are absent that otherwise should be present and what bony prominences should be easily felt but are not readily palpable) can be demonstrated to the patient's owner as part of the educational process to obtain agreement that the patient needs to lose weight.

BCS also can be used to estimate percent body fat. Studies have shown the correlation between BCS and percent body fat to be highly significant for pets with 45% body fat or less ($r^2 = 0.92$).[18] Percent body fat for ideal BCS (4 to 5/9 or 3/5) averages 20% and ranges from 15% to 25% of body weight. With the nine-point scale, each one-point change from ideal represents an increase or decrease of 5%. With the five-point

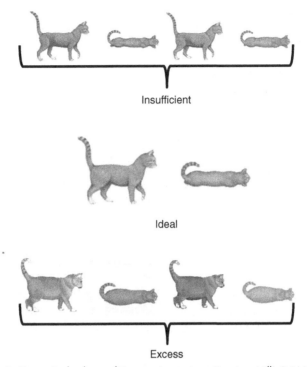

Insufficient

Ideal

Excess

Figure 2.4. Five-point body condition scoring system. Courtesy Hill's Pet Nutrition, Inc.

scale, each point represents a 10% change.[21,24,25] So if a pet has a BCS of 4/5, that correlates with approximately 30% body fat, and a BCS of 5/5 correlates with 40% (or more) body fat. Thirty percent body fat (BCS 4/5) is similar to the critical %BF in people, which marks an increased risk for ill effects from being overweight.

One limitation of these scales is that body fat percentage at the upper limits is not precise. Although a maximum percent body fat is assigned to the maximum BCS (5/5 or 9/9), in actual patients the degree of obesity varies. In reality, the maximum amount of body fat compatible with life is unknown and it is very likely many dogs and cats assigned a maximum BCS (5/5 or 9/9) have greater than the estimated 40% body fat.

A recent study documents that currently many dogs have body fat percentages of 50% or greater.[26] One aspect of this study was to compare the accuracy of using body fat percentages based on either the five- or nine-point BCS systems to dual energy X-ray absorptiometry (DEXA) scans to determine ideal body weight. DEXA scans of the 36 client-owned dogs weighing from 5 to 73.6 kg documented a mean body fat percentage of 45.9 in these patients (range 28.3% to 63.7%). While estimations of ideal body weight based on both BCS systems (5/5 and 9/9) were relatively accurate for dogs with less than 45% body fat, both BCS systems led to a significant over estimation of ideal body weight in dogs with greater than 45% body fat. This is important because 58% (21/36) of the dogs in this study were morbidly obese (more than 45% body fat based on DEXA). In this study use of BCS to estimate ideal body weight and consequently food dose would have resulted in recommending excess calories in more than half of these patients (Figure 2.5).

Underestimation of percent body fat and resultant overestimation of ideal weight may be a common cause for ineffective weight loss programs in extremely obese patients. One solution to this problem is to adopt a scheme similar to the obesity classifications in people using BMI. In this expanded system, the maximum BCS (5/5) is further categorized into subcategories 5 (a,b,c), which better define the degree of obesity (Table 2.3).[27] Using these subcategories may improve the

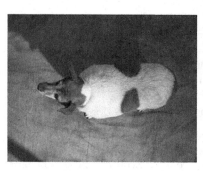 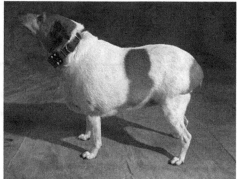

Figure 2.5. Many overweight patients are greater than 45% body fat. In this 16.8-kg female spayed Rat Terrier, BCS 5/5 or 9/9 estimates body fat at 35% to 45%. A dual energy X-ray absorptiometry analysis = 64% body fat. Photo courtesy of Dr. Angela Lusby.

Table 2.3. Classification scheme for BCS and degrees of obesity in pets.

Class	BCS	% Body Fat
Very thin	1	<5%
Underweight	2	10%
Normal	3	20%
Overweight	4	30%
Obese	5(a)	40%
Very obese	5(b)	50%
Extremely obese	5(c)	≥60%

Adapted from Toll PW, Yamka RM, Schoenherr WD, et al. Obesity. In: Hand MS, Thatcher CD, Remillard RL, et al., eds. *Small Animal Clinical Nutrition*, 5th ed. Topeka, KS: Mark Morris Institute, 2010;501–535.

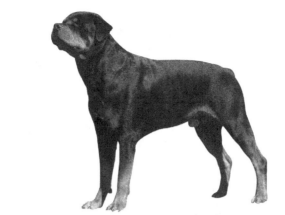

Rottweilers with a BCS of 5/9
have actual body fat **higher**
than the predicted 25%.

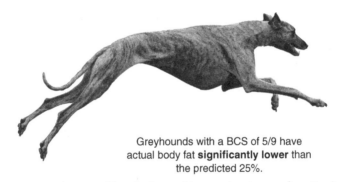

Greyhounds with a BCS of 5/9 have
actual body fat **significantly lower** than
the predicted 25%.

Figure 2.6. Muscle mass affects body condition scoring. Images from Fotolia.com.

accuracy of the estimation of ideal weight in very obese and extremely obese patients. Correctly selecting an ideal weight is the crucial first step in weight management programs because it determines the amount of food to feed these patients for weight loss.

Another caveat to using BCS to estimate percent body fat is breed variations. Muscle mass affects perception of BCS (Figure 2.6). One study using dual energy X-ray absorptiometry to determine body fat percentage in a limited number of purebred dogs documented this effect.[28] In this study, Greyhounds had a higher muscle mass than other breeds such that those judged to have a BCS of 5/9 had an actual body fat of 7.2%, significantly lower than the predicted 25% based on BCS scoring. Additionally, in these Greyhounds, each one-point change in BCS from ideal represented an increase or decrease of 1.5% body fat compared to the "normal" 5%. On the other end of the spectrum, Huskies and Rottweilers with a BCS of 5/9 had body fat of 31% and 32%, respectively, both higher than the predicted 25%. Increased age also affects BCS because lean muscle mass typically decreases with age. As a result, an older dog with a BCS of 5/9 may have a higher percent body fat than a younger adult dog.

If body condition scoring is to be used appropriately, these caveats must be taken into consideration. Additionally, body weights and body condition score must be recorded concurrently at each visit. Accurate historical data is one method of determining ideal body weight.

Weight at Maturity

Weight at the time the dog or cat reaches adulthood often is a good indicator of optimal weight, particularly if concurrent body condition assessments are available. However, weight at maturity may not be optimal if the animal was underfed or overfed during growth. The record of a body weight at the first adult visit may be meaningless unless accompanied by an assessment of body condition score. Time to maturity also varies. For most dogs and cats, maturity occurs around 12 months of age; however, giant-breed dogs may require up to 18 months to reach mature adult weight.

Breed Standards

For purebred dogs, determining ideal weight from published optimal weights by breed often is not accurate enough for an individual. Most breed standards list a wide range of weights. Based on data from the American Kennel Club, female Labrador Retrievers could weigh between 55 and 70 lbs and males between 65 and 80 lbs, an approximately 25% range in weight. If this method is used to estimate ideal weight, using the lower limit of the range will likely result in a more successful weight loss program.

Morphometric Measurements

Morphometry, the study of the mathematical and statistical properties of shape, has been used to estimate percent body fat. For people, BMI, which is based on morphometric measurements, is routine and practical. However, despite its routine use in people, BMI is influenced by differences in bone size and muscle mass.

Morphometry requires the use of some combination of measuring devices (e.g., a measuring tape, calipers) to measure different parts of the animal's body. Once the measurements are obtained, an equation is used to convert the morphometric measurements into estimates of percent body fat. For veterinary patients the diversity of body types, particularly among dog breeds, makes validating these equations problematic and to date has limited the usefulness of this technique.[27] In addition, equations validated for dogs may not be accurate in cats. Fat is deposited in slightly different body sites in cats compared to dogs. Cats store most of their fat subcutaneously along their ventral abdomen, in their faces, and intra-abdominally. Dogs deposit significant amounts of fat intra-abdominally and subcutaneously in thoracic, lumbar, and coccygeal areas. Even with these challenges, methods for morphometric analysis of dogs and cats have been reported.

To date, these methods should be considered semiquantitative because the measurements used to calculate percent body fat can vary considerably. Differences in measurements may result from:

1. Variations in coat thickness
2. Operator variability (i.e., tension on the tape measure)
3. Operator variability in determining the precise location of anatomic landmarks for measurement
4. Patient restraint, particularly in cats

Despite these challenges, and because they are designed to provide a specific, somewhat objective estimate of % BF, morphometric measurements may be of value in client communication.[29]

In a 2004 study the following gender-specific and gender-nonspecific equations in dogs were tested.[18]

Gender-specific formulas:

Males: (% BF) = −1.4 (HS in cm) + 0.77 (PC in cm) + 4

Females (% BF) = −1.7 (HS in cm) + 0.93 (PC in cm) + 5

Gender-nonspecific formulas:

$$\%BF = (-0.0034\,[\text{HS in cm}]^2 + 0.0027\,[\text{PCcm}]^2 - 1.9)/\text{BWkg}$$

In these equations HS is the height at the shoulder measured in centimeters and PC is the pelvic circumference at the level of the flank measured in centimeters.

Reasonable correlation existed between the % BF calculations using gender-specific and gender-nonspecific equations and the % BF as determined by DEXA. Height at the shoulder and pelvic circumference were the major determinates in all of these equations. Because pelvic circumference measurements change most with weight gain in the dog, using this site in the calculations is recommended by the authors of this paper but they caution that because of the variations in body types among breeds, these measurements may not always correlate well with % BF.

Furthermore these measurements may not be applicable to morbidly obese patients. The client-owned dogs in this study all had less than 40% body fat as determined by DEXA. Further studies comparing dogs of differing conformations and with greater than 40% body fat are warranted. In separate studies the following equations have been proposed and validated on limited populations:

Puppies: % BF $= 38.369 - 0:064$ (BMI)

Cats: % BF $= 66.715 - 0:061$ (BMI)

Dogs: % BF $= -12.937 + 0:696$ (AG)

where body mass index (BMI) is measured as L^2/W, length (L, cm) is measured from the nose to the base of the tail, weight (W) is measured in kilograms, and abdominal girth (AG) is measured as the circumference at the fifth to sixth lumbar vertebrae.[29]

To date, the lack of validation of these measures across a variety of dog and cat breeds limits their widespread use in clinical practice. However, recent work with morphometric measurements in dogs and cats may provide a validated mechanism that can be applied to all breeds and body types.

One study in 36 client-owned overweight or obese dogs (28% to 64% body fat based on DEXA) has led to the development of several regression equations for the prediction of lean body mass from body size data.[30] The best equations using the morphometric measurement data resulted in a $r^2 = 0.99$ and a predictability of 100% ($\pm$10%) using eight variables, including body weight. This approach holds great potential for the development of simple and accurate tools that can be used in clinical practice to determine ideal body weight. Further studies are ongoing to validate the equations and develop the tools for use in both dogs and cats.

Why Ideal Body Weight Matters

An accurate estimate of the patient's ideal weight is critical for a successful weight loss program. Veterinarians must accurately assess energy needs to prescribe appropriate food doses. If the starting point for these calculations (ideal body weight) is inaccurate, then the weight loss program is destined to fail. A key, often overlooked fact is that as weight increases because of increased percent body fat, an equivalent increase in calories needed for maintenance does not occur. Lean body mass uses calories; fat mass stores excess calories (Figure 2.7).

Consider, for example, a dog weighing 37.5 lb. If this dog is in ideal body condition he has 20% body fat. The resting energy requirement required to maintain lean body mass at this ideal body condition is 580 calories/day. As this dog gains body fat, this requirement does not change, despite the increase in body weight. This relationship is illustrated in Figure 2.7. If this same dog presented weighting 75 lbs, 45 of those pounds would be fat. Those 45 pounds of fat require little to no calories to maintain and should not be factored into the calculations for food dose.

Many veterinarians suggest selecting an "interim" target weight for morbidly obese animals. If this strategy is used in the previous example, the program will likely fail. Based on the RER for 50 lbs, the owner will

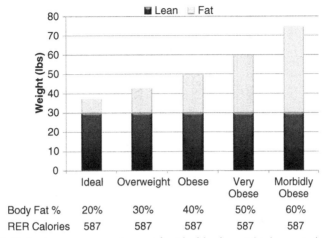

| Body Fat % | 20% | 30% | 40% | 50% | 60% |
| RER Calories | 587 | 587 | 587 | 587 | 587 |

Figure 2.7. Resting energy requirement for ideal body weight does not change with increased weight from increased % body fat.

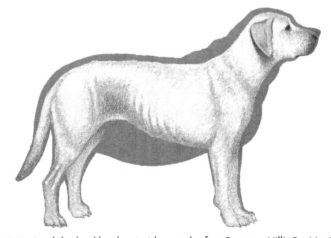

Figure 2.8. Feed the healthy dog inside, not the fat. Courtesy Hill's Pet Nutrition, Inc.

feed 741 calories/day, approximately 160 calories more than is required to maintain the ideal lean body mass (580 calories/day) and likely more than the dog is currently consuming to maintain the obese body condition. Remember, feed the healthy dog inside, not the fat (Figure 2.8).

Establish an Ideal Weight

Currently, all of the clinical tools for assessing body condition are relatively subjective. As a result, deciding the optimal weight for an individual patient can be problematic for the veterinarian and the pet owner, especially if the two disagree. Until more accurate methods are

Table 2.4. Estimating ideal body weight. Relationships between body condition score (BCS, five-point system) and actual body weight, ideal body weight, resting energy requirement (RER, kcal metabolizable energy [ME]/day), and estimated percent body fat (% BF). Actual body weight and BCS can be used to estimate a patient's ideal weight and associated RER, which can be further used to determine the amount of food to feed for weight loss.

Body weight (lbs)

BCS												
5	4.4	5.5	6.6	7.7	8.8	9.9	11	12.1	13.2	14.3	15.4	16.5
4	3.74	4.62	5.72	6.6	51.48	8.58	9.46	10.34	11.22	12.32	13.2	14.08
3	3.3	4.18	5.06	5.72	6.6	7.48	8.36	9.02	9.9	10.78	11.66	12.32
RER	95	112	129	144	160	174	189	203	216	230	243	256

Body weight (lbs)

BCS												
5	17.6	18.7	19.8	20.9	22	23.1	24.2	25.3	26.4	27.5	28.6	29.7
4	15.18	16.06	16.94	17.82	18.92	19.8	20.68	21.78	22.66	23.54	24.42	25.52
3	13.2	14.08	14.96	15.62	16.5	17.38	18.26	18.92	19.8	20.68	21.56	22.22
RER	268	281	293	305	317	329	341	352	364	375	386	397

Body weight (lbs)

BCS												
5	30.8	31.9	33	34.1	35.2	36.3	37.4	38.5	39.6	40.7	41.8	42.9
4	26.4	27.28	28.38	29.26	30.14	31.02	32.12	33	33.88	34.98	35.86	36.74
3	23.1	23.98	24.86	25.52	26.4	27.28	28.16	28.82	29.7	30.58	31.46	32.12
RER	408	419	430	441	451	462	472	483	493	503	513	524

Body weight (lbs)

BCS												
5	44	46.2	48.4	50.6	52.8	55	57.2	59.4	61.6	63.8	66	68.2
4	37.62	39.6	41.58	43.34	45.32	47.08	49.06	50.82	52.8	54.78	56.54	58.52
3	33	34.76	36.3	38.06	39.6	41.36	42.9	44.66	46.2	47.96	49.5	51.26
RER	534	553	573	293	612	631	650	668	687	705	723	741

Body weight (lbs)

BCS												
5	70.4	72.6	74.8	77	79.2	81.4	83.6	85.8	88	90.2	92.4	94.6
4	60.28	62.26	64.02	66	67.98	69.74	71.72	73.48	75.46	77.22	79.2	81.18
3	52.8	54.56	56.1	57.86	59.4	61.16	62.7	64.46	66	67.76	69.3	71.06
RER	759	777	794	812	829	846	863	880	897	914	931	947

Body weight (lbs)

BCS												
5	99	103.4	107.8	112.2	116.6	121	127.6	134.2	140.8	147.4	154	160.6
4	84.92	88.66	92.4	96.14	99.88	103.62	109.34	115.06	120.78	126.28	132	137.72
3	74.36	77.66	80.96	84.26	87.56	90.86	95.7	100.76	105.6	110.66	115.5	120.56
RER	980	1013	1045	1077	1108	1139	1186	1231	1277	1321	1365	1409

BCS	% BF
5	≥40
4	30
3	20

Example: A 70-lb dog has a BCS of 4/5. What is the ideal weight and associated RER and the approximate % BF?

1. Find the closest value for the dog's current body weight (69.74) in the row for BCS 4/5.
2. Locate the corresponding body weight for BCS 3/5 (ideal weight) in the row for BCS 4/5.
3. Below the ideal body weight of approximately 61 lbs, find the RER value for that weight, in this case 846kcal/day.
4. At the current BCS (4/5), the dog's approximate % BF is 30.

Adapted from Toll PW, Yamka RM, Schoenherr WD, et al. Obesity. In: Hand MS, Thatcher CD, Remillard RL, et al., eds. *Small Animal Clinical Nutrition*, 5th ed. Topeka, KS: Mark Morris Institute, 2010;501–535.

available, one way to provide an objective estimate is to use a table based on current BCS (Table 2.4). Locate the patient's body weight for its current BCS and read the corresponding body weight for its ideal BCS (3/5) from the table. This type of tool may be particularly helpful if there is a discrepancy between the veterinary health care team and the owner's perceived ideal body weight. This table is based on the assumption that a body condition score of 5/5 is equivalent to approximately 40% body fat. If patients are judged to have greater than 40% body fat, basing calculations on the information in Table 2.3 may be more accurate. If in doubt, assume the ideal body weight is less rather than more.

Gain Commitment

"Given that most parents of overweight children fail to recognize that their child has a weight problem, pediatricians should develop strategies to help these parents correct their misperceptions. Before instructing parents about dietary and exercise regimens, clinicians must first verify that parents know when they have a child with a weight problem and why they need to be concerned."[4] Substitute owners for parents and pet for children and this quote is equally applicable to veterinarians. Owners must be involved in weight loss and obesity prevention programs. However, for these programs to be successful the veterinary health care team must facilitate owner awareness of obesity. Lack of awareness has been cited as one of the main problems with managing obesity in clinical veterinary practice.[25]

One way for the veterinary health care team to demonstrate the importance of assessing body condition and determining ideal weight is to treat these procedures with the same significance as other diagnostic tests (e.g., heartworm tests, routine blood chemistry and urinalysis screening). Body weight and body condition assessment must be performed, recorded, and discussed with the owner at every visit. Recording an abnormal body condition score without verbally discussing the finding and its ramifications is futile. Few veterinarians would recommend and perform heartworm tests or routine screening blood chemistry and urinalysis without discussing the results with the owners, regardless of the results. If owners are to understand the health risks associated with abnormal body condition, veterinary health care teams must treat the diagnosis of this disease with the same emphasis as any other abnormal laboratory test result (Figure 2.9). After all, if owners are not being alerted that their pet is overweight, overweight pets will not receive appropriate treatment. Only when an owner perceives that their pet's weight is a problem will they be likely to employ changes to correct the problem.

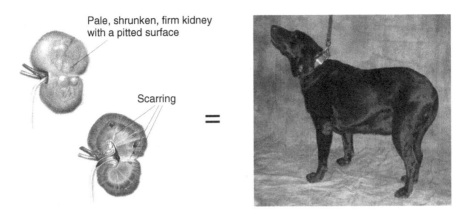

Figure 2.9. Abnormal body condition scores are as clinically important as abnormal laboratory findings. Courtesy Hill's Pet Nutrition, Inc.

Summary

The first step to a successful weight loss program is diagnosis of the disease. A variety of diagnostic tests are available. Pick one and use it consistently with every patient at every visit. The second step to a successful weight loss program is to determine the pet's ideal body weight. An accurate ideal body weight must be used for food dose calculations to produce effective weight loss. Using current (overweight) body weight to calculate daily calorie intake for weight loss generally leads to overestimation of daily food dose. Body condition scoring is the most widely used method of assessing body composition and can be clinically useful. It is important to remember that all of the current systems for BCS overestimate ideal body weight if pets have greater than 45% body fat. This overestimation of ideal body weight leads to insufficient caloric restriction for weight loss in these patients and frustration for both the owner and the veterinary health care team.

In Practice

Albert Einstein is credited with this definition of insanity: doing the same thing over and over again and expecting different results. This concept is particularly applicable to health care teams that continue to use weight loss programs that have failed in the past. One key component of failing weight loss programs may be the failure to correctly identify the pet's ideal body weight, which leads to erroneous calculations of calorie intake required to achieve weight loss. The following three examples demonstrate why reassessing how you determine ideal body weight may improve the success of your weight loss programs and stop the insanity.

Determine the ideal body weight and resting energy requirement for each patient using the five point body condition scoring system and Table 2.4.

Case 1: A 10-year-old Male Neutered German Shepherd weighing 113 lbs (Figure 2.10)

Body condition score:___
Ideal body weight:___
RER for ideal body weight:___

Case 2: A 7-year-old Male Neutered Golden Retriever Weighing 99 lbs (Figure 2.11)

Body condition score:___
Ideal body weight:___
RER for ideal body weight ___

Case 3: An 8-year-old Male Neutered Shih Tzu Weighing 21 lbs (Figure 2.12)

Body condition score:___
Ideal body weight:___
RER for ideal body weight:___

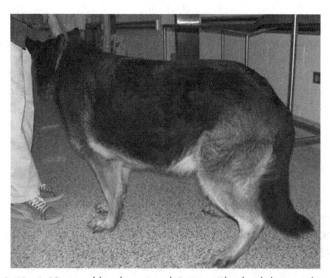

Figure 2.10. A 10-year-old male neutered German Shepherd dog weighing 113 lbs. Courtesy Hill's Pet Nutrition, Inc.

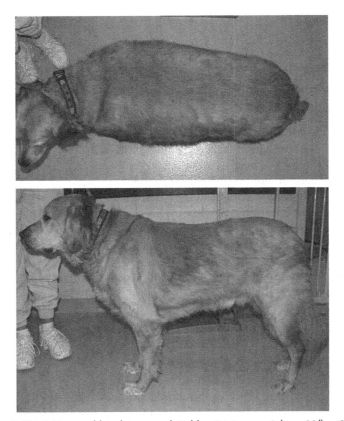

Figure 2.11. A 7-year-old male neutered Golden Retriever weighing 99 lbs. Courtesy Hill's Pet Nutrition, Inc.

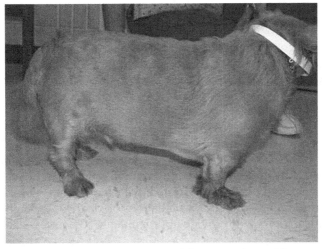

Figure 2.12. An 8-year-old male neutered Shih Tzu weighing 21 lbs. Courtesy Hill's Pet Nutrition, Inc.

Answers:

Case 1: 10-year Old Male Neutered German Shepherd Weighing 113 lbs

Body condition score: 5/5
Ideal body weight based on current BCS: 84 lbs
RER for ideal body weight based on BCS: 1,077
Actual percent body fat (DEXA): 43%
Ideal body weight based on % BF: 84 lbs
RER for ideal body weight based on % BF: 1,077
Because this dog's actual percent body fat did not exceed 45%, estimations of ideal body weight based on BCS are accurate.

Case 2: 7-year-old Male Neutered Golden Retriever Weighing 99 lbs

Body condition score: 5/5
Ideal body weight based on current BCS: 74 lbs
RER for ideal body weight based on BCS: 980
Actual percent body fat (DEXA): 50%
Ideal body weight based on % BF: 62 lbs
RER for ideal body weight based on % BF: 854
Excess calories from BCS based ideal weight: 126/day
This dog's actual percent body fat exceeded BCS estimations by only 5%, yet BCS based calculations provide about 15% excess calories/day. Weight loss programs based on this ideal body weight will not be successful.

Case 3: 8-year-old Male Neutered Shih Tzu Weighing 21 lbs

Body condition score: 5/5
Ideal body weight based on current BCS: 15.6 lbs
RER for ideal body weight based on BCS: 305
Actual percent body fat (DEXA): 59%
Ideal body weight based on % BF: 10.8 lbs
RER for ideal body weight based on % BF: 230
Excess calories from BCS based ideal weight: 75/day
It may be hard to imagine that a dog can have greater than 50% body fat. Sadly, this is much more common today than in years past. This owner will likely be frustrated by lack of success with a weight loss program based on BCS calculations of ideal body weight. BCS based calculations will provide approximately 33% excess calories/day.

References

1. Flegal KM, Carroll MD, Ogden CL, et al. 2010. Prevalence and trends in obesity among US adults, 1999–2008. *JAMA* 303:235–241.

2. Ogden CL, Carroll MD, Curtin LR, et al. 2007–2008. Prevalence of high body mass index in US children and adolescents. *JAMA* 303:242–249.

3. Towns N, D'Auria J. 2009. Parental perceptions of their child's overweight: An integrative review of the literature. *J Pediatr Nurs* 24:115–130.

4. Etelson D, Brand DA, Patrick PA, et al. 2003. Childhood obesity: Do parents recognize this health risk? *Obes Res* 11:1362–1368.

5. Ma J, Xiao L, Stafford RS. 2009. Underdiagnosis of obesity in adults in US outpatient settings. *Arch Intern Med* 169:313–314.

6. Riley MR, Bass NM, Rosenthal P, et al. 2005. Underdiagnosis of pediatric obesity and underscreening for fatty liver disease and metabolic syndrome by pediatricians and pediatric subspecialists. *J Pediatr* 147:839–842.

7. Lund EM, Armstrong PJ, Kirk CA, et al. 2006. Prevalence and risk factors for obesity in adult dogs from private US veterinary practices. *Intern J Appl Res Vet Med* 4:177–186.

8. McGreevy PD, Thomson PC, Pride C, et al. 2005. Prevalence of obesity in dogs examined by Australian veterinary practices and the risk factors involved. *Vet Rec* 156:695–702.

9. Holmes KL, Morris PJ, Abdulla Z, et al. 2007. Risk factors associated with excess body weight in dogs in the UK. *Journal of Animal Physiology and Animal Nutrition* 91:166–167.

10. Lund EM, Armstrong P, Kirk CA, et al. 1999. Health status and population characteristics of dogs and cats examined at private veterinary practices in the United States. *Journal of the American Veterinary Medical Association* 214:1336–1341.

11. German AJ, Morgan LE. 2008. How often do veterinarians assess the body-weight and body condition of dogs? *Vet Rec* 163:503–505.

12. Allan FJ, Pfeiffer DU, Jones BR, et al. 2000. A cross-sectional study of risk factors for obesity in cats in New Zealand. *Prev Vet Med* 46:183–196.

13. Singh R, Laflamme DP, Sidebottom-Nielsen M. 2002. Owner perceptions of canine body condition score. *J Vet Intern Med* 16:362.

14. Colliard L, Ancel J, Benet JJ, et al. 2006. Risk factors for obesity in dogs in France. *J Nutr* 136:1951S-1954S.

15. Colliard L, Paragon BM, Lemuet B, et al. 2009. Prevalence and risk factors of obesity in an urban population of healthy cats. *J Feline Med Surg* 11:135–140.

16. Freeman LM, Abood SK, Fascetti AJ, et al. 2006. Disease prevalence among dogs and cats in the United States and Australia and proportions of dogs and cats that receive therapeutic diets or dietary supplements. *J Am Vet Med Assoc* 229:531–534.

17. NIH. 1998. National Institutes of Health Obesity Education Initiative Expert Panel on the Identification, Evaluation, and Treatment of Overweight and Obesity in Adults: The Evidence Report. September.

18. Mawby DI, Bartges JW, d'Avignon A, et al. 2004. Comparison of various methods for estimating body fat in dogs. *J Am Anim Hosp Assoc* 40:109–114.

19. Armstrong PJ, Lund EM. 1996. Changes in body composition and energy balance with aging. *Veterinary Clinical Nutrition* 3:83–87.

20. Scarlett JM, Donoghue S, Saidla J, et al. 1994. Overweight cats: Prevalence and risk factors. *Int J Obes Relat Metab Disord* 18 Suppl 1:S22–28.
21. Laflamme DP, Kealy RD, Schmidt DA. 1994. Estimation of body fat by body condition score (abstract). Twelfth Annual Veterinary Medical Forum, American College of Veterinary Internal Medicine 985.
22. Laflamme DP, Schmidt DA, Deshmukh A. 1995. Correlation of body fat in cats using body condition score or DEXA (abstract). Thirteenth Annual Veterinary Medical Forum, American College of Veterinary Internal Medicine 1029.
23. Laflamme DP. 1993. Body condition scoring and weight maintenance. North American Veterinary Conference 290–291.
24. Laflamme DP. 1997. Development and validation of a body condition score system for cats: A clinical tool. *Feline Practice* 25:13–18.
25. Laflamme DP. 1997. Development and validation of a body condition score system for dogs: A clinical tool. *Canine Practice* 22:10–15.
26. Lusby AL, Kirk CA, Toll PW, et al. 2010. Effectiveness of BCS for estimation of ideal body weight and energy requirements in overweight and obese dogs compared to DXA (abstract). *Journal of Veterinary Internal Medicine* 24:717.
27. Toll PW, Yamka RM, Schoenherr WD, et al. 2010. Obesity. In: Hand MS, Thatcher CD, Remillard RL, et al., eds. *Small Animal Clinical Nutrition*, 5th ed. Topeka, KS: Mark Morris Institute, 501–535.
28. Jeusette I, Greco D, Aquino F, et al. 2010. Effect of breed on body composition and comparison between various methods to estimate body composition in dogs. *Res Vet Sci* 88:227–232.
29. Laflamme DP. 2006. Understanding and managing obesity in dogs and cats. *Vet Clin North Am Small Anim Pract* 36:1283–1295, vii.
30. Toll PW, Paetau-Robinson I, Lusby AL, et al. 2010. Effectiveness of morphometric measurements for predicting body composition in overweight and obese dogs. *Journal of Veterinary Internal Medicine* 24:717.

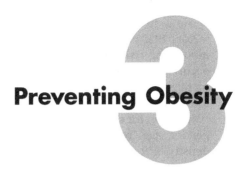

Preventing Obesity

Mark A. Brady, DVM, DACVECC

Basic Advice for Owners

Imagine how you would feel if you just found out that your doctor knew that you had a preventable disease that would shorten your life span, but she had avoided discussing this topic with you because she did not want to hurt your feelings. Would you be OK with losing five, 10, or 15 years due to this disease? Most people would be angry or at the very least confused by this action. Many would ask, "Why doesn't my doctor care about my well being?" Now imagine that your doctor reads this discussion and becomes very angry because she is adamant that she has had this discussion with you. The problem, according to her, is that you just don't listen to the recommendations she has provided. This lack of effective communication happens every day in veterinary offices regarding obesity.

We all understand that life has a beginning and an end; obesity just hastens the journey. Overweight and obese patients are common in veterinary medicine and their numbers are growing at a rapid rate. Treatment of obesity is sometimes analogous to trying to stop an avalanche once it has begun. There are many interrelated factors that contribute to the problem. However, the primary contributing factor involves inappropriate feeding practices by pet owners. Modifying this behavior can be a challenge and is discussed in the remaining chapters. The goal of this chapter is to aid in the development of a program to prevent obesity that can be applied to every patient presented to the veterinary health care team.

Practical Weight Management in Dogs and Cats, First Edition. Edited by Todd L. Towell.
© 2011 John Wiley and Sons, Inc. Published 2011 by John Wiley & Sons, Inc.

How do you prevent a disease? First we must understand the risk factors that contribute to the development of obesity. Eliminating or modifying risk factors may alter the course or prevent a disease from occurring. An example of this is the widely held belief that smoking increases the risk of developing lung cancer. The chances of developing this disease are decreased if you do not smoke. What are the potential risk factors for obesity? Several have been identified including genetics, gender, age, reproductive status, physical activity level, and caloric density of food (Table 3.1).[1,2]

Four areas should stand out as potentially modifiable. The most obvious is caloric density of the food. This may sound simple, but actually it encompasses a variety issues including the owner's feeding practices, the emotional connection between food and love, and the addition of treats and/or supplements to the main diet. A nutritional assessment of each patient that presents to the veterinary health care team is critical to controlling caloric intake (Table 3.2). This assessment provides information that can be used to create a nutritional plan for the pet owner. As the pet ages and/or activity levels or reproductive status changes, this plan must be adjusted to ensure that calorie intake remains appropriate.

While it may not be possible to change the reproductive status of the pet, it is critical that owners understand the impact gonadectomy has on calorie requirements. Gonadectomy significantly decreases the calories required to maintain a normal body weight. Continuing to feed pets the same amount of calories that maintained a healthy weight pre-

Table 3.1. Risk factors for obesity.

Risk factor	Modifiable?
Genetics	No
Age	No
Physical activity level	Yes
Gender	No
Reproductive status	Yes
Caloric density of food	Yes
Owner perceptions of body condition	Yes

Table 3.2. Nutritional assessment.

Complete medical/dietary history
Physical exam findings
Laboratory analysis
Key nutritional factors
Calculate caloric intake

surgery will likely lead to weight gain post surgery, a fact that is seldom communicated to pet owners. Teaching owners to perform body condition scores on their pets can help them identify weight gain before it becomes severe. Finally, the physical activity of a patient can directly affect it ability to maintain an ideal weight. Encouraging owners to incorporate exercise into a pet's daily routine will enhance weight management programs.

Nutritional Plan

The importance of developing a nutritional plan for healthy patients cannot be underestimated. Increasingly, clients are taking an active role in developing their own nutritional plans for their pets and many are choosing unconventional diets (e.g., raw, holistic, organic, all meat, etc). The veterinary team can have a strong influence on the nutritional choices clients make for their pets.

Clinical nutrition is not a static process. Nutritional requirements change over time or in the presence of disease. Life stage nutrition is the concept of providing a food designed to meet the optimal nutritional needs of a patient at a specific age or physiologic state. Life stage nutrition recognizes that feeding either below or above optimal nutrient levels can negatively affect biologic performance and/or health. The nutritional needs of an 8-week-old puppy, a 3-year-old neutered adult, and a 15-year-old geriatric dog are not the same (Figure 3.1). Performing

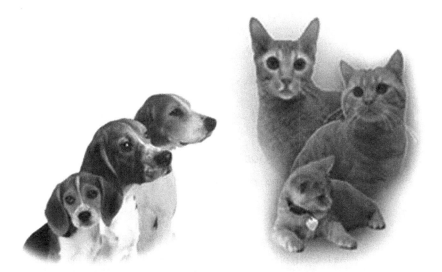

Figure 3.1. Life stage nutrition. Provide food designed to meet the optimal nutritional needs of a patient at a specific age or physiologic state. Courtesy Hill's Pet Nutrition, Inc.

a nutritional assessment at each visit is the key to ensuring pets are receiving the appropriate nutrition for their life stage.

Nutritional Assessment

In healthy pets, the nutritional assessment process helps identify risk factors for obesity. Once risk factors are identified, the feeding plan can be adjusted to include instructions to prevent this disease process from developing. After all, an ounce of prevention is worth a pound of cure. Performing a nutritional assessment is a two-step process, as illustrated in Figure 3.2. The first step involves assessment of the patient, food, and feeding method. The second step encompasses the development of a feeding plan and includes recommendations for food and feeding methods. This process is repeated at the next visit to determine the effectiveness of the feeding plan. The condition of the patient determines how often the plan is reassessed. The two-step process can be repeated any number of times, depending on the needs of each patient.

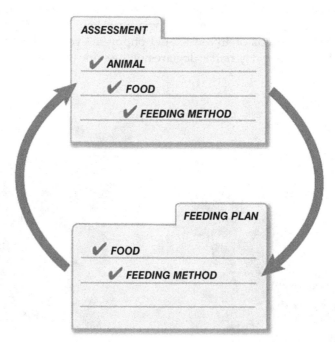

Figure 3.2. The two-step process of veterinary clinical nutrition. Used with permission from Thatcher CD, Hand MS, Remillard RL. Small Animal Clinical Nutrition: An Iterative Process. In: Hand MS, Thatcher CD, Remillard RL, et al., eds. *Small Animal Clinical Nutrition*, 5th ed. Topeka, KS: Mark Morris Institute, 2010;5.

Prevention of obesity can be accomplished by routinely assessing the patient and food, implementing a plan in which the nutrients and energy in the food are matched to the patient, and monitoring for long-term compliance or adjusting the recommendation when necessary. This should be completed each time a patient is seen at the hospital. Recording this information should be analogous to recording a temperature, pulse, and respiration in the medical record.

Step One: Assess the Current Situation

The Pet

The patient assessment is the first step in formulating a nutritional recommendation. The primary goal of this process is to identify the patient's nutrient needs. The patient assessment should include a complete medical and dietary history along with the veterinarian's complete physical examination. Proper interpretation of this information leads to a logical diagnostic workup. An accurate medical and dietary history is essential. A review of the medical record should provide objective historical information regarding the pet's previous health status, health maintenance procedures, and previously prescribed foods and/or medications. This information should be evaluated to determine if any of these historical factors are related to the pet's current nutritional status.

Even during routine wellness checks, a dietary history should include questions about the pet's weight, appetite, and recent therapies that may affect appetite or nutrient metabolism. A description should be obtained from the owner regarding the current feeding plan including the pet's food, feeding method, and eating/drinking habits. Carefully record all dietary facts such as type and brand of food, nutritional supplements, snacks, treats, table food, and amounts fed each day.

Medical records also provide clues about risk factors such as age, gender, neuter status, environment (e.g., multi-pet household), and medical/surgical problems (e.g., torn cranial cruciate ligament). Frequently reviewing this information permits early nutritional intervention for treatment of established malnutrition (e.g., obesity development) and for prevention in individuals at risk.

A thorough physical examination by the veterinarian can help define a pet's nutritional status as well as identify a disease process that may have a nutritional component. The examination should take the same form as the history taking: body system by body system. Assessment of body condition score (BCS) should be included in the physical exam. It is critical that a BCS be recorded in the medical record during each and every examination of the pet.

Anthropometry is the science that deals with body measurements, such as height, weight, and proportions. In humans, anthropometry is used to determine body mass index (BMI). Zoometrics or morphometric measurements are equivalent animal terms describing the same process. Body weight is the most common technique used in small animal medicine. However, in many pets, estimating an ideal body weight is difficult. Breed standards can provide some guidance but individual variation within breeds and mixed breed pets presents a challenge. Medical records provide valuable information about the pet's weight over time. In general, a good rule of thumb is that dogs and cats should weigh no more in later years than they did during their first full year of maturity.

> **Key Point**
>
> Cats and dogs should weigh no more in later years than they did during their first full year of maturity.

In some cases, the history and physical examination may suggest that a more in-depth work-up is required. This may include comprehensive blood work and/or ancillary diagnostic procedures. While no single laboratory test or other diagnostic procedure can accurately assess a patient's nutritional status, a biochemical profile, complete blood count, and urinalysis can provide insight into the presence of metabolic disorders and other disease processes that may benefit from a change in nutrition. Proper interpretation of this information allows the health care team to classify the nutritional problem and determine key nutritional factors that should be addressed.

Determining the key nutrients of concern and their target levels is fundamental to the formulation of a nutritional plan. The Association of American Feed Control Officials (AAFCO) publishes recommended nutrient profiles for dog and cat foods, which are the official source for nutrient information for dog and cat food in the United States. The values published by AAFCO are deemed adequate to meet the known nutrient needs of healthy dogs and cats. AAFCO makes recommendations for lower limits for all nutrients and upper limits for certain nutrients. These recommendations underscore the importance of providing nutrients in quantities that prevent inadequacies while not over supplementing some because excesses may be harmful to the pet.

Identifying key nutritional factors (KNF) for an individual pet can greatly simplify the approach to developing a nutritional plan. Because most commercial pet foods sold in the United States provide at least AAFCO allowances of all nutrients, if a commercial food is fed, the health care team only has to understand and focus on delivering the target levels of a few nutrients for a particular disease process. For

Table 3.3. Factors that affect key nutritional factors (KNFs) target levels.

Life stage
Physiologic state
Environmental conditions
    Temperature
    Housing
    Pet-to-pet competition
Underlying disease conditions or injury
Known losses through skin, urine, GI tract
Interaction of medication and nutrients
Ability of body to store certain nutrients
Interrelationships of various nutrients

obesity, the key nutritional factor is energy. Energy-supplying nutrients (e.g., fat, protein, and carbohydrates) should be controlled and non-energy-supplying nutrients (e.g., minerals, vitamins) increased to compensate for decreased daily caloric intake. Rather than having to assess all nutrients currently recognized for dogs and cats, we can focus on a diet that already provides these adjustments in KNFs. Several factors should be considered when determining KNFs and their target levels (Table 3.3). The factors that are important are determined on a case-by-case basis.

The Current Food

Obesity occurs when daily consumption of calories exceeds daily energy expenditure for a prolonged period. Several factors account for excessive caloric intake in pets. Owners prefer to buy foods that their pet eats readily. Therefore, most commercial foods are formulated to be highly palatable. Many commercial foods also are formulated to be calorically dense and highly digestible. The combination of highly palatable foods that are calorically dense served in oversized portions or free choice is a recipe for obesity. When formulating a nutritional plan it is crucial to evaluate the current food, keeping in mind the KNFs for obesity prevention, primarily calorie content. Evaluation of the current food can be performed in three steps: assess the nutritional adequacy statement, determine the dry matter nutrient content, and compare KNFs of the current food with the desired values for prevention of obesity.

Nutritional Adequacy Statement

The nutritional adequacy statement should be evaluated to determine whether the food has undergone AAFCO feeding trials or if it has been formulated to meet the nutrient requirements of a given life stage. This is an important point of differentiation. All pet foods sold in the United

States, with the exception of products clearly labeled as "treats" and "snacks" or "supplements," must contain a statement and validation of nutritional adequacy on the label. If a food is labeled "complete and balanced," "100% nutritious," or something similar, manufacturers must indicate the method and life stage that was used to substantiate this claim.

There are three methods used to substantiate claims: formulations, feeding trial, and family. The formulation method requires that the manufacturer substantiate a "complete and balanced" claim by calculating the nutrient content of the food using standard nutrient information about ingredients or chemical analysis of the final product. This method does not require the product to be fed to animals prior to offering it for sale. The formulation method is less expensive and less time-consuming than the other methods, but has been criticized because it does not account for acceptability of the food or nutrient availability.

The feeding trial method requires that the manufacturer perform a feeding trial following AAFCO protocols using the food as the sole source of nutrition. The feeding trial method is generally considered the preferred method for substantiating a claim.

The family method allows a manufacturer to perform a feeding trial on the lead member of a product family, then use analyses to ensure that other members of the product meet nutrient requirements. The family method is generally used to substantiate claims when a single formulation is offered in a variety of flavors. Examples of how to interpret nutritional adequacy statements are provided in Table 3.4.

These foods can be further subdivided into all-purpose and life stage foods. By regulation, all-purpose foods are formulated to meet the highest potential need (usually growth and reproduction). As a result, many KNFs that are appropriately high for growth and reproduction are excessive for adult maintenance. This is particularly true for calorie content. All-purpose foods tend to have a higher calorie content because they must meet the increased demands of growth and reproduction. Therefore, all-purpose foods may not be appropriate for pets prone to obesity. Life stage foods are formulated to provide an optimal amount of nutrients for a specific age or physiologic state. The nutritional adequacy statement on life stage foods indicates that the product is appropriate for one life stage, either growth and reproduction or adult maintenance.

Nutrient Content

Next, determine the food's dry matter nutrient content, focusing on key nutritional factors. This can present a challenge. Although all pet food manufacturers are required to include minimum percentages for crude protein and crude fat and maximum percentages for crude fiber and moisture on the label as part of the guaranteed analysis, other KNFs may not be listed. Guarantees are expressed on an "as is" or "as-fed"

Table 3.4. Interpreting nutritional adequacy statements.

Label claim	Interpretation	Recommended use
"Best Ever Beef Flavor Dog Food is formulated to meet the nutritional levels established by the AAFCO (Association of American Feed Control Officials) Dog Food Nutrient Profiles for maintenance of adult dogs."	This food has been formulated to meet the nutrient levels in the AAFCO Dog Food Nutrient Profile for adult maintenance. This product does not meet the nutrient profile for growth/lactation and has not undergone AAFCO feeding tests.	Life stage: Adult maintenance
"Animal feeding tests using the AAFCO procedures substantiate that Best Ever Lamb Meal and Rice Formula Dog Food provides complete and balanced nutrition for the growth of puppies and maintenance of adult dogs."	This food has successfully completed an AAFCO minimum protocol feeding trial for growing puppies (10 weeks of feeding) or is a family member of a tested product.	All purpose; adult maintenance and growth
"Best Ever Cat Food with Tuna provides complete and balanced nutrition for kittens and adult reproducing queens as substantiated by feeding tests performed in accordance with procedures established by the Association of American Feed Control Officials (AAFCO)."	This cat food (or a family member) has undergone AAFCO minimum protocol feeding studies for gestation/lactation and growth. This food is nutritionally adequate for adult cats but is not recommended by this manufacturer for long-term maintenance of adult cats. The language of the statement is not in compliance with AAFCO regulations.	Life stage: Growth and reproduction
"Animal feeding tests using the AAFCO procedures substantiate that Best Ever Chicken Flavor Dog Food provides complete and balanced nutrition for all life stages of the dog."	This dog food (or a family member) has undergone AAFCO minimum protocol feeding trials for gestation/ lactation and growth.	All purpose; growth, gestation/lactation, and maintenance

Adapted from Roudebush P, Dzanis DA, et al. 2010. Pet Food Labels, Table 9.6. In: Hand MS, Thatcher CD, Remillard RL, Roudebush P, and Novotny BJ. *Small Animal Clinical Nutrition.* Topeka, KS: Mark Morris Institute: 199.

basis. It is important to remember to convert these guarantees to a dry matter basis when comparing foods with differing moisture content. For example, consider two canned products with the following guaranteed analysis:

Product A

- Crude protein minimum: 12%
- Crude fat minimum: 18%
- Crude fiber maximum: 2%
- Moisture maximum: 72%

Product B

- Crude protein minimum: 12%
- Crude fat minimum: 18%
- Crude fiber maximum: 2%
- Moisture maximum: 82%

Do these products contain the same amount of protein? If not, which is higher in protein? To answer these questions the foods must be compared on a dry matter basis. Dry matter is the food remaining after water content has been removed. Using dry matter basis allows the amount of nutrients in the food to be compared without the dilution effect of water (Figure 3.3). This is particularly important when comparing dry foods to canned foods, but also when comparing moist products. Subtle differences in moisture content of moist products can result in marked differences in dry matter content and therefore the nutrient content of a given pet food. Remember, the dry matter content of the food contains all of the nutrients except water.

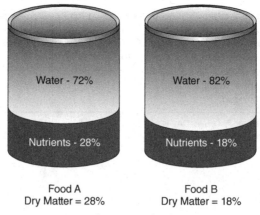

Figure 3.3. Dry matter content of two moist foods.

To answer our questions, the following calculations must be completed:

- Dry matter = 100% – moisture maximum (%)
  Product A dry matter = 100% – 72% = 28%
  Product B dry matter = 100% – 82% = 18%

- Dry matter basis (DMB) = % nutrient as fed/% dry matter × 100
  Product A = 12%/28% × 100 = 43% protein DMB
  Product B = 12%/18% × 100 = 67% protein DMB

Despite the fact that the guaranteed analysis of both products indicates a minimum protein of 12%, the difference in water content (dilution) means that Product B has significantly more protein on a dry matter basis than Product A. Figure 3.4 demonstrates the difference between DMB and as fed when comparing dry vs. moist foods. A moist product with a guaranteed analysis of 10% protein as fed actually contains more protein on a dry matter basis than a dry food with a guaranteed analysis of 20% protein.

For pets prone to obesity, the most important KNF is the calorie density of the food. Contrary to other KNFs of interest, calorie content should be compared on an as-fed basis. Currently in the United States, manufacturers are not required to include a statement of calorie content

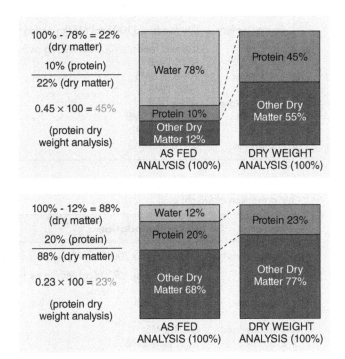

Figure 3.4. Comparing dry and moist moods on a dry matter basis.

on the label of all foods. At this time, it is only required for "light" and "less calorie" pet foods, but is voluntary on others.

If the statement is present it must be separate from the guaranteed analysis and appear under the heading "Calorie Content." The statement is based on kilocalories of metabolizable energy (ME) on an as-fed basis and must be expressed as kilocalories/kilogram (kcal/kg) of product. The statement also may be expressed in a more useful fashion, such as kilocalories/familiar household measure (e.g., kcal/cup, kcal/can), in addition to, but not in lieu of, the kcal/kg value. For nutrients of interest or calorie contents that are not listed on the product label, it may be necessary to contact the manufacturer. Manufacturer's addresses and toll-free phone numbers can be found on the product label. Many manufacturers provide online resources or printed keys which supply, among other things, the average nutrient contents of all of their foods listed on an as-fed, dry matter, and as-fed calorie basis.

Key Nutritional Factors

Last, compare the food's key nutritional factors with recommended levels for prevention of weight gain (Tables 3.5 and 3.6). Although

Table 3.5. Key nutritional factors (KNF) for dog foods labeled for prevention of weight gain.

KNF	Recommendation
Energy density	Dry foods: ≤3,100 Kcal ME/kg as fed
	Canned foods: ≤900 Kcal ME/kg as fed
Fat	≤14% DMB
Crude fiber	10–20% DMB
Protein	≥18% DMB
Carbohydrate	≤55% DMB
L-Carnitine	≥300 ppm DMB
Sodium	0.2–0.4% DMB
Phosphorus	0.4–0.8% DMB

Table 3.6. Key nutritional factors (KNF) for cat foods labeled for prevention of weight gain.

Factor	Recommendation
Energy density	Dry foods: ≤3,200 Kcal ME/kg as fed
	Canned foods: ≤950 Kcal ME/kg as fed
Fat	≤18% DMB
Crude fiber	15–20% DMB
Protein	≥35% DMB
Carbohydrate	≤40% DMB
L-Carnitine	≥500 ppm DMB
Sodium	0.2–0.6% DMB
Phosphorus	0.5–0.8% DMB

calorie content is the primary KNF for obese-prone pets, other nutrients of concern include L-carnitine, sodium, and phosphorous content. Avoiding excesses of phosphorous and sodium may be important in pets prone to obesity with risk factors for kidney disease. Similarly, avoiding excesses of magnesium, phosphorous, and calcium may be important in cats at risk for forming uroliths.

Feeding Method

How a client feeds his pet is a critical and often overlooked factor in obesity prevention. There are three typical methods for providing food: free-choice feeding, food-restricted meal feeding, or time-restricted meal feeding. Free-choice feeding, also known as *ad libitum*, means that more food than the pet will consume is always available. Pets can eat as much as they want, whenever they choose. With food-restricted meal feeding, the pet is given a specific quantity of food at each meal; ideally, the amount is based on caloric needs. Time-restricted meal feeding occurs when the pet is given an unlimited ration of food but is only allowed to eat for a set period of time. For many dogs this is equivalent to free-choice feeding. Most Labrador Retrievers can consume large volumes of food in a very short time.

Which of these methods is most popular? Which of these methods is most likely to promote obesity? The answer to these questions is the same: free-choice feeding. This is particularly true for cats. One study documented that 40% of owners provide food *ad libitum* for their cats.[3] The same study found that while the majority of dogs are fed one to two times/day, 30% also received "people food" and 40% got one or more commercial treat/day. The amount of food provided at each meal was not assessed.

Free-choice feeding may appear to have advantages compared to the other feeding practices. This method is convenient for the pet owner but is limited to dry foods. It ensures adequate food availability and mimics natural feeding behavior, allowing a pet to eat several times throughout the day. In multi-pet households, less dominant animals have a better chance at getting their share of food. However, the problem with this feeding method is that it is difficult to monitor appetite and food intake. As a result, over consumption leads to weight gain. From the standpoint of obesity prevention, pet owners should be discouraged from using the free-choice feeding method. If a pet owner is unwilling to modify this feeding method, a calorie-restricted food is the best long-term food option.

Food-restricted meal feeding is the best option for obesity prevention if portion sizes are appropriate. Portion control is critical to preventing obesity. In America, portion sizes served at many restaurants have grown exponentially over the last 20 to 30 years. This is one of the factors leading to the growing trend of obesity in people. The idea that

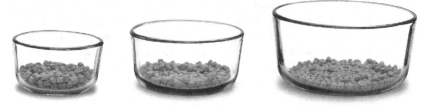

Figure 3.5. Difference in appearance of 1 cup (8 oz) of dry kibble in three bowl sizes.

a meal should be super sized has altered the perception in many homes as to what is a normal portion.

It is reasonable to believe that pet owners have a difficult time assessing normal portion sizes for their pets. Excessive portion sizes mean pets have the opportunity to consume excess calories. Food-restricted meal feeding facilitates monitoring of appetite and food intake and better control of body weight provided portion sizes are controlled. The reluctance of some pet owners to adopt this feeding method may relate to perceived lack of convenience and increased labor involved. Some owners may find it hard to accept smaller portion sizes, which they may view as "depriving" their pet. Feeding pets in small containers may help owners limit the amount of food offered at each meal. Visual cues are important to people; the same amount of food can look like a lot or a little depending on the size of the bowl (Figure 3.5).

Time-restricted meal feeding is of limited usefulness in dogs and has little if any practical application in cats. Many dogs can eat an entire meal in less than two to three minutes. Cats are often unwilling to eat immediately after food is offered. This method provides inaccurate control of food and is very labor intensive. Similar to free-choice feeding, this method increases the risk for obesity because of the inability to control food intake.

A combination of methods is sometimes preferred by pet owners, particularly when a combination of canned and dry food is used. Typically in this situation, the canned food is offered in a food-restricted manner while the dry food is provided free choice. This option is common in many households across America. The problems with this method are similar to those discussed above. Primarily, food intake is difficult to monitor, which generally leads to over consumption of calories and weight gain/obesity.

Step Two: Specific Nutritional Recommendation

Owners deserve and expect a specific recommendation from the veterinary health care team on how to prevent obesity in their pets. Despite the proliferation of information available on the Internet and recommendations from paraprofessionals (groomers, breeders, etc.) the veterinary health care team is still the most frequently cited and trusted source of information about pet nutrition.[3] To be useful, a nutritional recommendation should include specific instructions on the type of food and feeding method that is most appropriate for the individual pet and pet owner circumstances.

Choosing a Food

For adult pets prone to obesity, there are typically three choices: adult maintenance foods, light foods, and therapeutic weight control foods. A thorough understanding of the benefits and limitations of each food type is vital to deciding which food is the best choice for a given patient.

Maintenance Foods

Maintenance foods make up the majority of products purchased in pet retail chains, grocery store, discount warehouses, and farm and feed stores. Maintenance foods are intended to be the sole source of nutrients, except water, for an adult dog or cat. Maintenance foods are an appropriate choice if the nutritional assessment demonstrates a pet with a normal body condition and ideal weight, and with limited risk factors for obesity. All-purpose maintenance foods, those labeled for all life stages or for growth and adult life stages should be avoided. These foods are by necessity be more calorie dense than those labeled specifically for adult maintenance, so over consumption of calories is more likely.

If the pet is obese-prone or slightly overweight (less than 15% above ideal body weight), pet owners may wish to reduce their pet's current food instead of switching to a calorie-restricted food. This approach is not recommended and is rarely successful for a variety of reasons. The primary reason is that by restricting calories to induce weight loss, the available nutrient intake also is being reduced. Commercial pet foods balance all other nutrients to the energy content of the food. Decreasing calorie intake decreases intake of other nutrients as well.[4]

Importantly, the digestibility and total energy extracted from a calorically dense food increases slightly when less is fed.[1] In essence, the body becomes more efficient at extracting as many nutrients and calories as possible, negating the benefit of reducing the amount fed. Finally, most maintenance diets are calorically dense, meaning they contain more fat than calorie-restricted foods. Fat has about 2.25 times the calories of an equivalent weight of carbohydrate or protein (Figure 3.6).[1,4]

Fat is a good source of energy because it is digested and metabolized very efficiently. In one study, dogs lost more weight and body fat when fed a low-fat, high-fiber food compared to one of equal calories that was high in fat and low in fiber.[5] Human studies have demonstrated that consumption of fat produces less thermic effect, meaning the

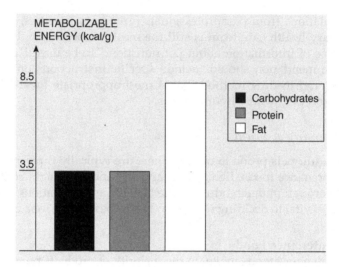

METABOLIZABLE
ENERGY (kcal/g)

8.5

3.5

■ Carbohydrates
■ Protein
□ Fat

Figure 3.6. Comparison of energy density of carbohydrates, protein, and fat.

postprandial metabolic energy expenditure is decreased, compared to ingestion of protein or carbohydrate.[6] Therefore, a calorie-dense food relying on fat as its primary energy source tends to support retention of body weight and body fat, even when total calories are reduced. For these reasons, a light or therapeutic obesity prevention food is indicated.

Restricted Calorie Foods: "Light" Foods

When should a "light" food be chosen for a patient? Several factors should be considered when deciding whether to use this type of food. First, does the pet possess any risk factors that may lead to obesity? Consider, as an example, the typical young indoor intact male cat in normal body condition that presents for an elective castration. What long-term food recommendation should be given to this client post surgery? This patient has multiple risk factors for obesity including gender (male), indoor housing, and gonadectomy.[7] This is an ideal candidate to recommend a light food for long-term maintenance.

Prevention of rebound weight gain after undergoing successful weight reduction is another indication for light food. This phenomenon has been demonstrated in humans, dogs, cats, and many other species.[5,6] Rebound weight gain is most extreme when weight loss is rapid, and is most common in dogs allowed access to an energy-dense food after weight reduction.[5] One option for minimizing rebound weight gain is for patients to make a transition from therapeutic weight loss foods to a light food once they have reached their target weight.

This is not as easy as it may sound. Pet foods marketed as restricted in calories can vary widely in caloric content. A recent study designed to determine the range of calorie density and feeding directions for

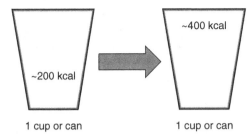

Figure 3.7. Commercial weight management foods are not created equal. There can be much as a two-fold difference in calorie density.

commercially available diets designed for weight management in dogs and cats found wide variations in calorie density.[8] Close to 100 foods marketed for weight management were easily identified. Marketing claims included weight loss, obese prone, to maintain healthy weight, avoid unwanted weight gain, lose excess weight, and reduced calorie. Given the availability of apparently suitable foods for pet owners to choose from, why it is so hard to maintain their pets at a healthy weight? The greater than two-fold difference in calorie density among these foods may be one explanation (Figure 3.7).

In the aforementioned study, calorie density for 44 canine diets ranged from 217 to 440 kcal/cup and from 189 to 398 kcal/can for moist foods. For the 49 feline diets, calorie density ranged from 235 to 480 kcal/cup for dry and from 78 to 172 kcal/can for moist foods. More than half of the foods (58%) had calorie densities on the basis of kcal/kg of diet that were greater than the AAFCO maximum calorie density for light foods, making weight maintenance or loss difficult without careful control of calorie intake. Controlling calorie intake is confounded by the wide range in feeding directions and high variability in estimates of calorie requirements for weight loss or maintenance provided on the labels of these products. These challenges highlight the importance of a specific nutritional recommendation from the health care team, which includes recommendation of a specific product, a specific amount of product to be fed, and specific instructions on offering the food (Figure 3.8).

Recommending foods that are specifically labeled light or "lean" may be helpful. AAFCO provides strict criteria for the terms "light," "lean," "reduced calorie," and "reduced fat" that must be met if the label contains these terms (Table 3.7). By definition, a food advertised as light, lite, or low calorie must be reduced in caloric density when compared to a maintenance food. The food label also must contain feeding directions that reflect a reduction in calorie intake consistent with the intended use.[9] If these two criteria are not met, then the food is not a light food.

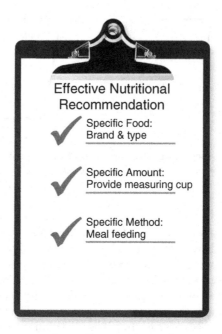

Figure 3.8. Components of an effective nutritional recommendation. Image from Fotolia.com.

Therapeutic Obesity Prevention Foods

The daily energy requirements necessary to maintain a healthy weight can vary significantly; some individuals may need less than 50% of the calories required by the average dog or cat to maintain a healthy weight (Figure 3.9). For these pets, commercially available weight management foods may not be appropriate.

If significant calorie restriction is required, it is important that the chosen food have an increased nutrient/calorie ratio to avoid restriction of essential nutrients. Therapeutic weight loss foods generally are not recommended for prevention of obesity. Therapeutic weight loss foods are discussed in Chapter 4. Therapeutic obesity prevention foods are specifically formulated to address this need. A limited number of these products are available through veterinarians (Table 3.8). For many obese-prone pets, therapeutic obesity prevention foods may be the best option, particularly if owners choose to continue free choice feeding. These products are generally less calorie dense than products available over the counter, so they may decrease the risk of pets gaining weight. However, no food, if consumed in excess will prevent obesity. The health care team should educate owners on how to assess body condition in their pets. If unintended weight loss or gain occurs with the use of these products, owners should consult the health care team. The amount of food offered may be adjusted accordingly or an alternative type of food may be indicated.

Table 3.7. Model Pet Food Regulation PF10 of the Association of American Feed Control Officials (AAFCO) defines limits and labeling requirements for claims related to restricted calorie and fat content. The regulation was implemented in the United States in January 1998.

Maximum calories or fat allowed for "light" or "lean" claims depending on moisture content and intended species*			
	Dry foods (<20% moisture)	Semi-moist foods (20–<65% moisture)	Moist foods (65% moisture)
Dogs			
Light (also "lite," "low calorie")	3,100 kcal ME/kg	2,500 kcal ME/kg	900 kcal ME/kg
Lean (also "low fat")	9% fat	7% fat	4% fat
Cats			
Light (also "lite," "low calorie")	3,250 kcal ME/kg	2,650 kcal ME/kg	950 kcal ME/kg
Lean (also "low fat")	10% fat	8% fat	5% fat

All values on as-fed basis
ME = metabolizable energy
*"Light" (or similar terms) on pet food labels must bear a calorie content statement as described in AAFCO PF9. "Lean" and "low-fat" pet food labels must bear a maximum percentage crude fat guarantee.
"Less" or "Reduced Calories"
For dog or cat food labels bearing a claim of "less calories," "reduced calories," or similar words, a maximum level of calories is not stipulated in the regulations. However, the percentage of reduction and the product of comparison must be explicitly stated on the label. The product label also must bear a calorie content statement, and feeding directions should reflect a reduction in calories compared with feeding directions for the product of comparison. Comparisons between products in different categories of moisture content are considered misleading.
"Less" or "Reduced Fat"
For dog or cat food labels bearing the claims of "less fat," "reduced fat," or similar words, a maximum percentage of fat is not stipulated in the regulations. However, the percentage of reduction and the product of comparison must be explicitly stated on the label. The product label also must bear a maximum crude fat guarantee immediately after the minimum crude fat guarantee in the mandatory guaranteed analysis information. Comparisons between products in different categories of moisture content are considered misleading.

Adapted from Toll PW, Yamka RM, et al. 2010. Obesity, Box 27.6. In: Hand MS, Thatcher CD, Remillard RL, Roudebush P, and Novotny BJ. Small Animal Clinical Nutrition. Topeka, KS: Mark Morris Institute: 513.

Rebound weight gain is a potential problem after discontinuing a therapeutic weight loss food. This is most likely to occur when a pet makes the transition to an energy-dense food and is fed free choice. The period immediately following successful weight loss is crucial. Owners should understand the importance of preventing rebound weight gain. Therapeutic obesity prevention foods are often the best choice for the immediate post weight loss period. Communication of these facts to an owner is paramount to preventing the recurrence of obesity in these pets.

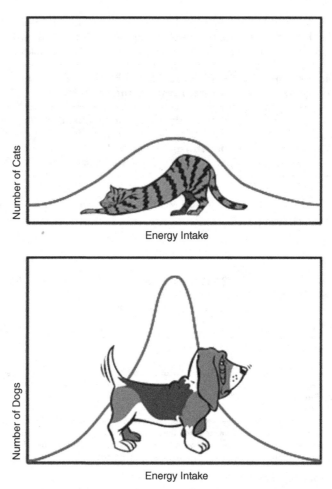

Figure 3.9. Average energy intake required to maintain a healthy body weight in dogs and cats. Courtesy Hill's Pet Nutrition, Inc.

Feeding Amounts

"I don't understand how my pet could be overweight; I followed the feeding instructions on the bag." Raise your hand if you ever heard that concern from one of your clients. This situation often leads owners and veterinary health care team members to conclude that all patients seem to get fat when eating a particular brand food. The problem with this conclusion is that it overlooks many factors that determine the energy requirement of each individual patient. In simplistic terms, the feeding guides and package labels we rely on to provide recommendations on how much to feed are analogous to throwing a dart at a dart board. In fact, you could think of the food quantity recommendations as highly

Table 3.8. Key nutritional factors for therapeutic obesity prevention foods.

Obesity prevention products for dogs	Form	Kcal/ kg (As fed)	Protein % (DMB)	Fat % (DMB)	Crude fiber % (DMB)
Hill's® Prescription Diet® w/d® Canine	Canned	890	17.9	12.7	12.4
AAFCO maximum calories for "light" canned foods		**900**			
Hill's® Prescription Diet® w/d® with Chicken Canine	Dry	2928	19.1	8.7	17.1
Hill's® Prescription Diet® w/d® Canine	Dry	2986	18.9	8.8	16.4
AAFCO maximum calories for "light" dry foods		**3100**			
Royal Canin Veterinary Diet™ Canine Weight and Stone WS30™ Small Breed Adult	Dry	3126	35.5	12.4	8
Iams® Veterinary Formula Weight Control D/Optimum Weight Control	Dry	3242	28.7	9.5	3
Royal Canin Veterinary Diet™ Canine Weight and Osteo WO28™ Large Breed Adult	Dry	3249	34.1	12.9	9.5
Obesity prevention products for cats					
Hill's® Prescription Diet® w/d® with Chicken Feline	Canned	811	39.6	16.6	10.6
AAFCO Maximun Calories for "light" canned food		**950**			
Hill's® Prescription Diet® w/d® with Chicken Feline	Dry	3187	39.9	9.9	7.6
AAFCO maximun calories for "light" dry food		**3200**			
Hill's® Prescription Diet® w/d® Feline	Dry	3227	39	9.8	7.6
Iams® Veterinary Formula Weight Control D/Optimum Weight Control	Dry	3503	38.6	12.2	1.5

scientific guesstimates. Calculated energy requirements should be used as guidelines, starting points, or estimates for individual animals, and not as absolute requirements.

A graph of the daily energy requirements for populations of dogs or cats is a bell-shaped curve (Figure 3.9). As mentioned, the energy intake of an individual dog or cat may vary by about 50% above or below the average requirements, even within the same age group. All estimates of energy needs and amount fed should be evaluated by body condition assessment and adjusted as necessary. Prevention of obesity should be an important goal of each feeding program for adult dogs and cats. Prior to continuing this discussion we should review some of the terminology used in discussing energy requirements.

Energy requirements can be expressed in several ways, depending on the physiologic and environmental condition in which the measurement is made. Basal energy requirement (BER) represents energy needs for a normal, awake, fasting, resting animal in a thermoneutral environment.[4] BER is also known as basal metabolic rate, basal energy expenditure, or fasting heat production.[4]

Resting energy requirement (RER) differs from BER in that the animal is not in a fasted state. RER represents the energy requirement for a normal animal at rest under thermoneutral but not fasted condition.[4] RER includes the energy needed for digestion, absorption, and metabolism of food as well as energy necessary to recover from previous physical activity. RER is sometimes referred to as resting energy expenditure.[4]

Maintenance energy requirement (MER) is the energy needed for moderate physical activity plus basal metabolism and the energy required to obtain, digest, and absorb food in amounts necessary to maintain body composition. MER does not include energy necessary to support additional activity such as exercise, work, gestation, lactation, or growth. Maintenance energy expenditure is another way of saying MER.

Daily energy requirement (DER) represents the energy necessary for physical activity (e.g., exercise, work, gestation, lactation, or growth) plus RER.[4] DER is dependent on the life stage and activity level of an individual. In practice, when estimating energy requirements of an individual, one of the following equations can be used:

$$RER = 70 \times (BW_{Kg})^{0.75}$$

$$RER = (30 \times BW_{Kg}) + 70$$

For practical purposes, resting energy requirements can be found in table form in many manufacturers' product keys, feeding guide software, and in Table 3.9. To determine the daily energy requirement, RER is multiplied by a factor based on physical activity estimates to calculate DER (Table 3.9). The amount of food is determined by dividing the estimated DER by the calories/cup or calories/can of the food. This is the amount of food the owner should provide per day.

Based on these definitions, there are multiple sources of potential errors when calculating energy requirements for dogs and cats. Do age,

Table 3.9. Resting energy requirements for dogs and cats.

Resting energy requirements		
lbs	kg	RER (kcal/day)
1	0.5	39
2	0.9	65
3	1.4	88
4	1.8	110
5	2.3	130
6	2.7	149
7	3.2	167
8	3.6	184
9	4.1	201
10	4.5	218
11	5.0	234
12	5.5	250
13	5.9	265
14	6.4	280
15	6.8	295
16	7.3	310
17	7.7	324
18	8.2	339
19	8.6	353
20	9.1	366
25	11.4	433
30	13.6	497
35	15.9	558
40	18.2	616
45	20.5	673
50	22.7	729
55	25.0	783
60	27.3	835
65	29.5	887
70	31.8	938
75	34.1	988
80	36.4	1037
85	38.6	1085
90	40.9	1132
95	43.2	1179
100	45.5	1225
105	47.7	1271
110	50.0	1316
115	52.3	1361
120	54.5	1405
125	56.8	1449
130	59.1	1492
135	61.4	1535
140	63.6	1577
145	65.9	1619
150	68.2	1661
155	70.5	1702
160	72.7	1743
165	75.0	1784

(Continued)

Table **3.9** *Continued*

Resting energy requirements		
lbs	**kg**	**RER (kcal/day)**
170	77.3	1824
175	79.5	1864
180	81.8	1904
185	84.1	1944
190	86.4	1983
195	88.6	2022
200	90.9	2061

Feline maintenance DER (kcal/day)
Normal, neutered adult = 1.2 × RER
Intact adult = 1.4 × RER
Geriatric = 1.1 × RER
Obese-prone adult = 1.0 × RER
Weight loss = 0.8 × RER

Canine maintenance DER (kcal/day)
Normal, neutered adult = 1.6 × RER
Intact adult = 1.8 × RER
Geriatric = 1.4 × RER
Obese-prone adult = 1.4 × RER
Weight loss = 1.0 × RER

activity level, environmental conditions, neuter status, breed, gender, or an underlying disease state effect energy requirements for a given patient? Yes, all of these factors can have an effect on the energy needs of an individual.

Does age affect energy requirements? A decrease in physical activity coupled with a loss of lean body mass (LBM) may affect energy requirements in geriatric dogs and cats. A loss of LBM would be expected to decrease the basal metabolic rate because muscle tissue has a high energy requirement. Some geriatric dogs and cats seem to spend an inordinate amount of time sleeping; therefore, their DER estimate is probably closer to their RER.

Calculations that have been developed to estimate RER in dogs and cats were based on pets in thermoneutral environments. However, in the real world, pets do not always live in controlled environments. Housing and climate changes should not be overlooked when evaluating energy requirements. Energy is used to dissipate heat when temperatures are above the thermoneutral zone. Conversely, when temperatures are below the thermoneutral zone, energy is used to maintain core body temperature. Individual characteristics of the animal including hair length, coat density, and subcutaneous fat deposition also affect the energy requirements in response to the environment.

Would you expect the energy requirement of a Saint Bernard to correlate with that of a Greyhound? Would an indoor-only domestic shorthair have the same requirements as an indoor/outdoor domestic shorthair of the same age, gender, and reproductive state? Does gender affect overall energy requirements? In people, the energy requirements of men are greater than women because of a proportionately greater muscle mass. However, this effect has not been found in dogs or even evaluated in cats.[4]

Because of the extraneous factors that may affect the energy requirements of an individual, it is important to remember that when you recommend a feeding amount to a pet owner, you are providing an estimate at best. Therefore, the amount fed will likely need to be adjusted over the course of an individual's life as a result of changes in any of these factors. Because of these variables, recommendations from the product label or feeding guide supplied by manufacturers are not accurate for every individual. Understanding this simple concept can go a long way toward obesity prevention in the hospital.

Measuring the food intake is the only way to know if any of these factors alter the energy requirements of an individual patient. The most accurate way to determine DER for an individual pet is to determine the total amount of calories consumed while the pet is maintaining an ideal body condition. Calorie densities for an extensive list of commercially available foods (dog and cat, canned and dry) are available on the Association for Pet Obesity Prevention website (www.petobesityprevention.com). If owners provide significant calories from "human" foods, these must be included in an estimate of daily energy intake. Calorie content of most foods can be found at www.nutritiondata.com. Needless to say, this is not always practical or even possible, but is worth the effort.

Key Point

Calculated daily energy requirements and label feeding guides are ESTIMATES. Amounts should be adjusted to maintain ideal weight.

Once all applicable variables have been taken into consideration, feeding amount recommendations should be based on the best available information, either current daily intake or calculated estimate of requirements. Don't forget that client education and the use of a standardized measuring cup are two of the most important aspects of obesity prevention. If the exact amount of calories consumed each day is unknown, adjusting the feeding plan becomes difficult. It is important to encourage clients to measure the quantity of food provided each day. This is the only way to answer the question, "How much should I be feeding my pet?"

How Should I Feed My Pet?

In an ideal world, every pet would be fed a food designed to meet their specific life stage and style in an amount that maintains ideal body condition. In the real world, the veterinary health care team should make a specific recommendation that includes the type of food, a specific amount, and instructions on how to provide the food. Meal feeding may not always be possible, but feeding strategies can be developed to minimize the chance of over consumption of calories. Some of these strategies are discussed in the following section on lifestyle considerations. Owners should be reminded that obesity may shorten their pet's life span. Client education regarding measurement of food quantity and monitoring of food intake allows adjustment of the feeding plan to maintain optimal body weight through the pets' life.

Life Stage and Lifestyle Considerations

Effect of Neutering

Gonadectomy should be considered a nutritional moment of truth. Cats and dogs undergoing elective ovariohysterectomy or neuter are at risk of becoming obese. Modifications of metabolic rate, feeding patterns, and body composition occur. These changes lead to an overall increase in body weight and body fat in both species. This section examines the evidence available and explains these changes and preventative measures that pet owners can use at home to maintain their pets' normal body condition.

> **Key Point**
>
> Gonadectomy is a nutritional moment of truth.

Several studies have evaluated the effect of gonadectomy on metabolic rate. Most have concluded that metabolic rate is decreased in neutered male and female cats compared to intact cats. An early study documented a decrease in metabolic rate, estimated by heat coefficient, of 28% in male cats and 33% in female cats.[10] Based on results of this study, to maintain a normal body weight, energy intake would need to decrease by about 30% after gonadectomy.[10] Another study demonstrated a 15% decrease in energy needed to maintain body weight in male and female cats after gonadectomy.[11] This result was only statistically significant for female cats.[11]

The decrease in metabolic rate after elective ovariohysterectomy and neuter is debated. Energy expenditure on a lean mass basis should not be significantly different after neutering. Because gonadectomy is not associated with loss of lean body mass, the basal metabolic rate should remain constant. However, a change in body composition (e.g., increase in body fat) related to modifications in feeding behavior may be a key driver to explain the reduction in metabolic rate.[12-14] Studies of female cats and dogs after gonadectomy document that to maintain an optimal body composition, reduction in energy intake of 15% to 40% was necessary in neutered female cats and 20% to 30% in neutered female dogs.[11,15,16] *Ad libitum* feeding is not recommended, particularly because the ability to self regulate food intake appears to be altered post gonadectomy.

Changes in feeding behavior resulting in increased body weight and body fat post gonadectomy have been documented in both dogs and cats. Over the short term, neutered cats seem to be unable to self-regulate their food intake.[12-15] Similarly, dogs appear unable to self-regulate their caloric intake after elective gonadectomy. A 59% increase in food consumption was noted in neutered female dogs fed a palatable food *ad libitum* for a period of four months.[16] Changes in body composition and increased body weight and body fat have been shown to result directly from an increase in caloric intake in cats.[12-15] Studies in dogs have demonstrated that after elective ovariohysterectomy or neuter a significant change in feeding behavior and activity level occurs. An increase in caloric intake secondary to increased food consumption occurs in female dogs after ovariohysterectomy.[17] A 20% increase in food intake after ovariohysterectomy was documented, compared to intact dogs fed *ad libitum*. A study of 591 client-owned dogs demonstrated increased body weight secondary to increases food intake after neutering in 42% of male and 32% of female dogs.[10] This study also documented a decrease in activity for neutered male and female dogs.

Free-choice feeding coupled with the inability to control intake leads to rapid increases in body weight and body fat in neutered pets.[12-18] In cats, changing to a low-fat, low-energy food helped reduce body weight gain compared to cats with access to a high-fat, high-energy food.[14] However, neither group of cats maintained normal body composition when fed *ad libitum*. Feeding a fixed amount of food to ovariohysterectomized dogs that were exercised regularly allowed them to maintain their body weight after surgery.[19] No similar study could be identified in cats.

Summarizing the evidence presented above, we can draw some conclusions regarding the effects of gonadectomy on pets. Neutering is a risk factor for the development of obesity in cats and dogs. Self-regulation of food intake is compromised in neutered cats and dogs. Voluntary consumption of food available free choice may increase as much as 50% in the months after neutering. If caloric intake is not controlled after gonadectomy, obesity will develop. This change in body composition and increased body weight and body fat increases the patient's risk for many health-related diseases (e.g., diabetes, cardiovascular or orthopedic disease, etc.) and shorten its life span.[10,20,21]

Key Point

Neutered pets are unable to self-regulate food intake. Consumption may increase by 50% post surgery.

How do we prevent this risk factor from causing obesity? The obvious answer would be to not perform elective ovariohysterectomy or neuter. The benefits of gonadectomy include controlling unwanted behaviors and unwanted reproduction, and reducing the risk of cancer and other diseases of reproductive organs.[22] Because development of obesity is easily controlled, for most pets these benefits outweigh the risk. Owners must understand that obesity is a preventable disease if calorie intake is controlled. Additionally, they must understand that they ultimately control the caloric intake of their pet. This fact cannot be debated or argued.

At discharge from elective gonadectomy, owners should be provided with a specific nutritional recommendation for their pet. Remember the energy requirement of individuals is highly variable, making it difficult to make a broad recommendation that includes every patient. However, controlling food intake and increasing exercise are recommendations that can apply to all pets. Development of a feeding plan based on the principles of a complete patient assessment and adjustment of that plan should be the cornerstone to prevent obesity. The reader is encouraged to use a client education handout to educate pet owners about the development of obesity post gonadectomy.

Multi-pet Household Feeding Strategies

The majority of families in America currently own a dog, a cat, or both, and 90% consider their pet a member of the family.[23] Therefore, it is critical that health care team members educate these owners on the proper feeding strategy for their four-legged family members. The feeding and social behavior of cats and dogs differ greatly, and these differences are important to understand when developing feeding strat-

Table 3.10. Feeding behavior of felines and canines.

Feline	Canine
Strict carnivore	Omnivore
10–20 meals/day	2–3 meals per day
Feed day and night	Feed during daylight
Frequent feeders	Glutton feeders
No social value in meal	Social value in meal

egies in multi-pet and multi-species households (Table 3.10). Cats are true carnivores, whereas dogs are omnivores. The nutritional needs for each species vary.

Cats in the wild typically eat 10 to 20 meals/day and prefer to eat alone. Feral cats must hunt day and night to consume sufficient food because each meal may contain as few as 30 kcal (estimated caloric content of a mouse). Importantly, observational studies show that feral cats often fail in their attempts to catch prey; in fact, only 13% of tracked prey is actually caught.[24] A significant amount of energy is expended in the process of obtaining food. This continuous hunting cycle, consuming small meals frequently throughout the day, also can be seen in house cats. Cats confined to indoors will hunt for food 10 to 20 times a day; unfortunately, they are rarely unsuccessful in obtaining food.

Dogs are considered opportunistic eaters and have developed anatomic and physiologic characteristics that permit digestion and usage of a variety of food types.[23] Domesticated dogs today typically have an abundance of food, and most dogs are solely dependent on their owners to provide their complete nutritional needs. Interestingly, humans and canines regard food and eating in a similar fashion, with an emphasis on social interaction vs. hunger. Humans and dogs are social animals and each tries to control the relationship, typically through the use of food (especially treats). Owners often anthropomorphize the relationship, which can lead to bad habits in the pet-owner relationship. For example, if dog owners satisfy a variety of requests for attention by giving food/treats, dogs quickly learn how to get that "yummy treat." This bad habit leads to ritual formation and ultimately to eating disorders/obesity.[25]

In typical households, the rhythm of food supply for pets depends on the owner's lifestyle. Two or three meals are often fed during the day: in the morning before going to work, in the evening when returning, and/or just before going to bed. The lifestyle preferences of owners must be taken into consideration when recommending a feeding program.

To begin developing feeding strategies for pets, the veterinary health care team, and the veterinary technician in particular, must obtain a detailed history, including a nutritional history, of each pet.

The nutritional history should include the feeding protocol (e.g., whether the pet is fed at designated meals or has free choice, the amount of food given, the family member responsible for feeding the pet), and the type or types of food given to the pet. The health care team should determine whether the pets receive supplements or medications and how much of each substance the pet consumes each day. Determining the number and species of pet(s) in the household is another crucial part of developing a feeding strategy. This may indicate access to foods not considered by the owner as part of the intended diet.

Cats

Meal-restricted feeding of individual pets is ideal but often not possible. Dogs are more likely to be meal fed. Cats are more likely to be free-choice fed. In multiple cat households, owners are often reluctant to separate each cat at feeding time. If providing food all day is important to the owner, the following feeding method will work for single or multiple-cat households.

1. Calculate the total amount of calories to be fed for the day. In multiple-cat households, add the calorie requirement for each cat to get the total "household" calories/day.
2. Determine whether cats are fed canned, dry or a combination of these foods on a daily basis.
3. If it is important for the owner to leave dry food available free choice but also provide canned food, then the following equation can be used to determine the amount of food to feed: DER/cat × number of cats = household calories; household calories/2 = calories per feeding; Calories/feeding × 0.25 = calories as canned; calories/feeding − calories as canned = calories as dry food.

For example: Your client has three cats, all between the ages of three and five years. Two have normal body condition scores but are considered obese-prone (12 lb and 10 lb), one is considered overweight (15 lbs, BCS 4/5). The DER for an obese-prone 10-lb cat is 1 × RER or 218 kcal/day. The DER for an obese-prone 12-lb cat is 1 × RER or 250 kcal/day. The estimated ideal weight for the 15-lb cat is 12 lbs. The DER for weight loss is 0.8 × RER for ideal body weight (0.8 × 250 kcal) = 200 kcal/day. The total/day for this household is 668 calories. The owner likes to meal feed canned food twice/day. One 3-ounce can of a light adult maintenance food contains 75 kcal. Twenty-five percent of the household calories is approximately 150 kcal. This can be divided into two feedings by splitting a 3-ounce can of food (approximately 25 kcal/cat/feeding) between the three cats morning and evening.

The remaining 520 calories are provided by a dry therapeutic obesity prevention food with a caloric density of 280 kcal/cup. The 1 and 3/4 cups of dry food are divided roughly in half. The smaller portion (3/4 cup) is distributed into multiple (5 to 6) small containers or treat balls in the morning, the remaining 1 cup in the evening. The containers are placed in varying locations throughout the house. Owners should be encouraged to place food bowls on different floors of the house, on shelves, behind furniture, etc. to engage hunting behavior. To decrease stress and competition, there should be at least one more feeding station (bowl or treat ball) than there are cats.

Hiding multiple food bowls/treat balls serves two purposes. First, no one cat can bully the other cats and guard the food. Second, this stimulates the cat's natural tendency to hunt for food, which provides environmental stimulation and a bit of exercise. This method is not appropriate if dogs also have access to the food. If dogs and cats occupy the same living space, food bowls for cats can be placed on elevated surfaces, out of the reach of dogs. Alternatively, cats and dogs can be restricted to separate areas (floors) of the house.

All food should be placed in a quiet, safe, secure place.[26,27] If the obese cat is fed food different from the normal weight cats, owners can place the normal cat's food where the obese cat cannot reach. If the obese cat cannot jump/ or climb, place the normal weight cat's food high. Alternatively, place the normal cat's food in a box with an opening too small for the obese cat, but large enough for the normal cat. If social conflicts arise among the housemates, then a cat or perhaps all cats need to be fed separately.

Another remedy is to feed the cats at the same time, but supervise the feeding and pick up all bowls when the cat finishes eating. In addition, owners must place the feeding bowls at a significant distance from the litter box(es) and sleeping areas (Figure 3.10).

Finally, cat owners must be educated about potential behaviors exhibited by cats that may increase the amount of caloric intake. Cats

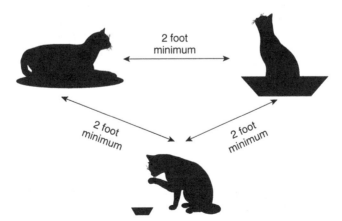

Figure 3.10. Minimum distance between feeding, sleeping, and toileting areas for cats. Images from Fotolia.com.

today are notorious for trying to solicit food from their owners when their bowl is empty. Cats have a learned behavior in which if they vocalize (cry, meow) and rub their human, the human will respond by filling the food dish. This learned behavior can lead to obesity. The health care team must educate owners to feed only the amount calculated and not reward the soliciting behavior with food. Instead, owners should use this signal to interact with their cat. Playing, grooming, and simply petting the cat, rather than food, are often a remedy to the affection the cat is seeking.[28] Furthermore, playing is a great way to increase exercise and help maintain an ideal body condition.

Dogs

Health care team members know that dogs are social animals and in today's society are considered members of the family. However, owners need to be educated about the feeding strategy for their dogs. Dogs relate to a hierarchy, in which it is typical for the human owner to be the alpha dog. If more than one dog is in a family, the hierarchy is established naturally. In the United States, 46% of dog owning families have more than one dog and many own more than one species.[23] As a new pet is introduced to the family, some dogs may show an increased interest in food, while others may not eat for a day or two. Often, jealousy arises over food, toys, beds, and even the owner. The hierarchy finds dogs raising the hair on their backs and withers in defense of their food bowl.

One consideration in multi-pet households is free-choice feeding, because dogs perceive there to be enough food for all and less dominant dogs have a better chance to get a share of the food provided.[25] Nevertheless, free-choice feeding is not recommended, especially if the more dominant dog ingests too many calories and the less dominant dog ingests too few calories. Both of these instances can lead to medical problems. The owner's interceding in the hierarchy often leads to dogs being fed separately. In households with more than one species, the bowls must be separated so one species cannot get the other's food. Again, a cat's food bowl may be placed high and out of reach of the dog. This is an important point to remember when counseling clients with multiple species in the home. Separating the dog food and the cat food helps to prevent aggression/protection behaviors as well as excessive caloric intake.

Clients also need to be reminded to watch the feeding of pets by children. Toddlers often drop food on the floor where both cat and dogs have free access. Older children may give in to the begging by their "four-footed siblings." These foods are not formulated for cats and dogs, and excess can lead to obesity and potentially other medical problems. The same is true in households that have other species. Avian pellets that fall out of the aviary are highly palatable to dogs. Horse feed is palatable, and often dogs and outdoor cats can be found helping themselves to horse feed. Health care team members must find out the complete family make-up as part of the nutritional history and educate clients regarding other foodstuffs their pet may be getting.

Considerations for Mature Pets

As pets age are they at risk for developing obesity? If so, what is the harm in maintaining this state? In answering this question it is important to remember that there is a large variation in health status between individual pets. Stated another way, chronological age (e.g., 7 years old) does not always match physiological age. Aging is not a disease, but it does make an individual more susceptible to underlying health issues.

A multitude of factors may play a role in the development of age-related disease processes. Some examples are breed size, genetics, nutrition, and environmental factors. The harm in maintaining this state of malnutrition is an increased risk in the development of several disease states that may decrease life expectancy, for example, the development of diabetes mellitus in cats. Identified risk factors in cats for this disease include age, gender, and obesity.

If we use diabetes mellitus as a model, we realize that there are potential complications and health implications with this individual that ultimately may affect quality of life and life expectancy. However, the problem is communicating this urgency to the pet owner to get him to act. In our diabetic example, is it effective to tell the owner that as his pet ages and maintains an overweight state it is at an increased risk of developing this disease? What if your client has no experience with diabetes? Do you think the ramifications of this disease process may be too difficult to comprehend? Might he ignore your advice because he does not understand the importance of your message? If the answer to this last question is yes, then we need to revisit the primary goal of having this conversation with our client. The desired outcome in this hypothetical scenario is either to get the client to feed the patient an appropriate caloric ration so that a normal body condition is maintained or undertake a weight management program that results in weight reduction back to a normal body condition.

To reach this desired outcome, we must first address the initial question posed at the start of this section. Are pets at risk for developing obesity as they age? More than 50% of dogs and cats 5 to 10 years of age are reported to be overweight or obese.[21] This means that about one of every four pets presenting to veterinary practices in this country has excessive body fat. Potential explanations for this include changes in energy requirements, decreases in lean body mass, and reduction in physical activity.

A decrease of 12% to 13% in the DER of dogs has been noted to occur at around seven years of age.[23] Additional studies in older dogs have drawn similar conclusions, but report changes in MER rather than DER.[21] Age-related energy requirements in older cats remain controversial. The author is unaware of any well-controlled studies that have been conducted to determine the energy needs of older cats. A primary driver of basal metabolic rate is lean body mass (LBM) because it contains the most metabolically active cells. Skeletal muscle, skin, and organs constitute LBM. Loss of LBM occurs in dogs and cats as they age.[21] Exercise helps to preserve LBM and also increases energy requirements. Again, as dogs and cats age there appears to be a decrease in physical activity, which reduces energy requirements. These interrelated factors lead to a state of reduced energy needs. If caloric intake is not adjusted, the patient is at risk of becoming overweight.

Two important facts emerge from this discussion. As pets age, they become more vulnerable to disease and susceptible to being overweight. Obesity may significantly increase the risk of developing certain diseases. These factors affect pets' quality of life and life expectancy. The majority of pet owners might identify with this core message. They cannot change the genetic make-up of their pet, species, sex, or breed. How do they improve their pet's quality of life and enjoy their companionship for as long as possible? They can control what they feed and how much. Maintaining an ideal body condition goes a long way toward reducing their pet's risk for disease and probably increases it's life span. Pet owners can increase the number of veterinary assessments per year, which allows monitoring of vital organ function and adjustment of the nutritional plan if necessary to maintain health.

Making Exercise a Part of Lifestyle

The health care team should encourage clients to exercise their pets frequently. Exercise is a necessary part of the pet's daily routine because it increases energy expenditure, reduces the loss of lean muscle mass, and maintains or improves RER. Exercise truly is the only practical means to create a deficit between energy taken in and energy used (Figure 3.11).

The average adult dog reaps health benefits from as little as 20 to 45 minutes of moderate exercise daily. However, an exercise plan for an out-of-shape pet (and owner) should begin slowly, with the activity level increasing gradually based on how much the pet can tolerate.[29] Start by recommending either a brisk five-minute walk with the pet or five minutes of rolling a ball across the yard for it to chase. This begins to increase the aerobic capacity of the dog and the owner with the ultimate goal of safely achieving 30 minutes of aerobic exercise.

Pets love to play and they want to play or interact with their owners. Owners should pay attention to what their pets are trying to tell them. Many unwanted behaviors in pets are the result of boredom

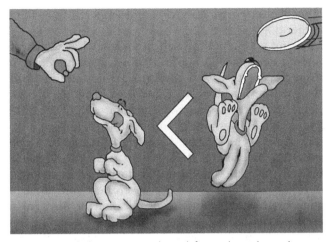

Figure 3.11. Exercise helps create a calorie deficit; calories burned are greater than calories consumed. Courtesy Hill's Pet Nutrition, Inc.

or stress. Exercise can alleviate boredom and relieve stress, both for pets and owners.

Some owners who may be reluctant to exercise their pets may be delighted to play with them. Exercise sounds like one more thing owners have to do, whereas finding time to play sounds more like something owners want to do. This subtle difference in communication style may make the difference for you client's pets. A useful resource for pet owners and health care team members is www.petfit.com. This site offers a variety of tools including the "Training Room" with Gunnar Peterson, personal trainer and dog lover. This site is supported by The American Veterinary Medical Association and Hill's Pet Nutrition's Alliance for Healthier Pets in an effort to raise awareness and provide solutions for the epidemic of pet obesity.

The veterinary health care team should encourage owners to engage in a variety of play activities that fit with the owner's lifestyle. Remember, asking an owner to dramatically change her behavior is much more challenging than increasing behaviors that are already part of her routine. Walking is simple, burns calories, and tones muscles. It also is a good way to get fit without jarring joints or muscles.[30] Swimming is another good exercise. It requires more calories than walking, so the same number of calories can be burned in a shorter amount of time.[1] Many breeds love the water, but remember that if the dog is not an avid swimmer, it should wear a safety jacket (flotation device). Throwing a ball for the dog to chase is a great activity for owners with any size yard. Playing fetch simulates many dogs' natural instinct to chase and retrieve prey. Dogs and humans love adventure, so consider recommending that your client take a hike with her dog. Local dog parks also offer excellent opportunities for well mannered dogs to run and romp with other dogs.

Exercising with a pet can be fun for the whole family. Children can and should get involved with the four-legged members of the family. Children can interact with pets in activities similar to those already mentioned. Families also can get involved in agility, flyball, Frisbee, and breed-specific activities such as herding. Many local 4-H programs provide opportunities for the entire family.

Many clinics offer doggie day care. This may be a good option for owners who are unable to increase their dog's exercise at home. Supervised interactions with other dogs increases daily activity and calories burned. If more controlled exercise is indicated, physical rehabilitation may be appropriate. Application of physical rehabilitation principles to weight loss in dogs is covered in Chapter 6. Regardless of the program, remind owners that the endurance of both the dog and the owner must be built gradually.

Cat owners must be more creative when trying to increase their pets' activity level. Fortunately, a variety of interactive toys (e.g., laser pointers, feather toys, noisy balls) are available to get cats moving and to increase the time they spend with their owners, thereby strengthening the human–animal bond. Owners also can take advantage of their cats' natural instinct to hunt prey. As discussed previously, owners can make cats hunt for food by hiding appropriate amounts in various bowls or dishes placed throughout the house, such as on bookshelves, on different floors of the house, and in hidden areas. This feeds (no pun intended) their natural hunting instinct while exercising. Providing food in cat treat toys encourages play and rewards the activity with food, even in the owner's absence. Many cats have been trained to walk on a leash. Again, walking is a great form of exercise for both the cat and owner and is a safe alternative for the indoor cat to be outdoors. The Ohio State University Indoor Cat Initiative website is an excellent resource for owners and health care teams: www.vet.ohio-state.edu/indoorcat. It includes information on increasing activity and nutrition recommendations.

Exercise should be an enjoyable activity that is fun for life, for both the pet and the pet owner. A study by the American Heart Association found that a person's life expectancy could increase by two years by burning 2,000 calories a week through exercise.[30] Another study published in the Journal of the American Veterinary Medical Association found that dogs lived almost two years longer than the control (overweight) group by being kept lean over their entire lives.[20] Exercise enriches the human-animal bond and lengthens the time we have with our pets.

Remind your clients that pets rely on them for their daily needs, and exercise is an important part of overall well being. Together, pets and owners can stay fit and have fun for a lifetime.

Conclusion

The bad news is that obesity is epidemic in our pets. Overweight pets have a shortened life span and are at risk for a variety of chronic diseases. The good news is that obesity is a preventable disease. Your job as a health care team member is to educate and work with owners to develop a specific nutritional plan for the lifelong health of their pets.

In Practice: The Case of the Automatic Feeder

A cat owner contacted me because her cat was having issues with his weight. At the time her 6-year old neutered male domestic shorthair cat weighed more than 25 lbs. He was an "only cat" and lived inside exclusively. The owner was currently feeding a good quality light dry food purchased at a pet retail chain, free choice. After completing a nutritional assessment, we discussed at length this cat's potential risk factors for obesity: indoor only, neutered male, and most of all free-choice feeding.

Key Points

- Neutered pets require 25% to 30% fewer calories
- Neutered pets do not self regulate food intake
- Free-choice feeding promotes over consumption
- Daily exercise is lacking

Specific Nutritional Recommendation

- Goal weight: 18 lbs
- Food: Therapeutic weight loss food (dry)(266 kcal/cup)
- Calculation: DER for weight loss = 0.8 × 339 (RER for 18 lb cat) DER = 271
- Amount: 1 cup dry therapeutic weight loss food/day
- How to feed: Owner purchased automatic feeder

Several feeding methods were discussed with the owner. She was not able to provide food in multiple sites throughout the apartment. She did purchase an automatic feeder that could be programmed to dispense 1/4 cup of dry food at approximately six-hour intervals (four times a day). Follow up weight checks were scheduled at monthly intervals.

After two months on the program, the cat had gained 1 lb of body weight. The owner, in an accusatory tone, insisted the food was not working; in fact it was making her cat fatter and I didn't know what I was doing. At this point it is only fair to let you know that this client also happened to be my sister. I responded as most brothers would, in an accusatory tone, that she must not be able to follow directions because I know the product works. Stop me if this sounds like a conversation you have had with a pet owner, hopefully without the sibling rivalry part. After we had both taken deep breaths, I recommended she observe her cat's eating habits over the weekend. I reinforced the amount of food he should be consuming: 1 cup of dry food/day. My sister contacted me the next week with an explanation. Her cat, smart boy that he is, had figured out how to insert his front paw into the door of the feeder and trigger the machine to dispense food. He could and did eat anytime he desired! Basically, he was feeding himself free choice. We brainstormed alternative methods of controlling intake and settled on providing 1/4 cup dry food in his bowl twice a day and filling a cat treat dispenser toy with 1/4 cup twice a day. She purchased a feather toy and promised to start playing with him in the evenings. At the next recheck he had lost 1.5 lbs and there was peace in the family.

References

1. Burkholder WJ, Toll PW. 2000. Obesity. In: Hand MS, Thatcher CD, Remillard RL, et al., eds. *Small Animal Clinical Nutrition, 4th Edition*. Topeka, KS: Mark Morris Institute, 401–430.
2. Laflamme DP. 2006. Understanding and managing obesity in dogs and cats. *Vet Clin North Am Small Anim Pract* 36:1283–1295, vii.
3. Laflamme DP, Abood SK, Fascetti AJ, et al. 2008. Pet feeding practices of dog and cat owners in the United States and Australia. *J Am Vet Med Assoc* 232:687–694.
4. Gross KL, Wedekind KJ, Cowell CS, et al. 2000. Nutrients. In: Hand MS, Thatcher CD, Remillard RL, et al., eds. *Small Animal Clinical Nutrition 4th Edition*. Topeka: Mark Morris Institute, 20–107.
5. Roudebush P, Schoenherr WD, Delaney SJ. 2008. An evidence-based review of the use of therapeutic foods, owner education, exercise, and drugs for the management of obese and overweight pets. *Journal of the American Veterinary Medical Association* 233:717–725.
6. Laflamme DP. 2006. Understanding and managing obesity in dogs and cats. *Veterinary Clinics of North America: Small Animal Practice* 36:1283–1295.
7. Scarlett JM, Donoghue S, Saidla J, et al. 1994. Overweight cats: Prevalence and risk factors. *Int J Obes Relat Metab Disord* 18 Suppl 1:S22–28.
8. Linder DE, Freeman LM. 2010. Evaluation of calorie density and feeding directions for commercially available diets designed for weight loss in dogs and cats. *J Am Vet Med Assoc* 236:74–77.
9. AAFCO. 2008 Official Publication: Association of American Feed Control Officials.
10. Jeusette I, Nguyen P, Diez M. 2005. Neutering: Can obesity be avoided. Proceedings 15th ECVIM-CA Congress 108–111.

11. Hoenig M, Ferguson DC. 2002. Effects of neutering on hormonal concentrations and energy requirements in male and female cats. *American Journal of Veterinary Research* 63:634–639.

12. Kanchuk ML, Backus RC, Calvert CC, et al. 2002. Neutering induces changes in food Intake, body weight, plasma insulin and leptin concentrations in normal and lipoprotein lipase-deficient male cats. *J Nutr* 132:1730S–1732.

13. Martin L, Siliart B, Dumon H, et al. 2001. Leptin, body fat content and energy expenditure in intact and gonadectomized adult cats: A preliminary study. *Journal of Animal Physiology and Animal Nutrition* 85:195–199.

14. Nguyen PG, Dumon HJ, Siliart BS, et al. 2004. Effects of dietary fat and energy on body weight and composition after gonadectomy in cats. *American Journal of Veterinary Research* 65:1708–1713.

15. Harper EJ, Stack DM, Watson TDG, et al. 2001. Effects of feeding regimens on bodyweight, composition and condition score in cats following ovariohysterectomy. *Journal of Small Animal Practice* 42:433–438.

16. Jeusette I, Detilleux J, Cuvelier C, et al. 2004. *Ad libitum* feeding following ovariectomy in female Beagle dogs: Effect on maintenance energy requirement and on blood metabolites. *Journal of Animal Physiology and Animal Nutrition* 88:117–121.

17. Houpt KA, Coren B, Hintz H. 1979. Effect of sex and reproductive status on sucrose preference, food intake, and body weight of dogs. *J Am Vet Med Assoc* 174:1083–1085.

18. Jeusette I, Daminet S, Nguyen P, et al. 2006. Effect of ovariectomy and *ad libitum* feeding on body composition, thyroid status, ghrelin and leptin plasma concentrations in female dogs. *Journal of Animal Physiology and Animal Nutrition* 90:12–18.

19. Le Roux P. 1983. Thyroid status, oestradiol level, work performance and body mass of ovariectomised bitches and bitches bearing ovarian autotransplants in the stomach wall. *J South Afr Vet Assoc* 54:115–117.

20. Kealy RD, Lawler DF, Ballam JM, et al. 2002. Effects of diet restriction on life span and age-related changes in dogs. *Journal of the American Veterinary Medical Association* 220:1315–1320.

21. Laflamme DP. 2005. Nutrition for aging cats and dogs and the importance of body condition. *Veterinary Clinics of North America: Small Animal Practice* 35:713–742.

22. Chun R, Garrett L. 2005. Urogenital and Mammary Gland Tumors. In: Ettinger S, Feldman EC, eds. *Textbook of Veterinary Internal Medicine Diseases of the Dog and Cat, 6th Edition.* St. Louis: Elsevier Saunders, 784–789.

23. Debraekeleer J, Gross KL, Zicker SC. 2000. Normal Dogs. In: Hand MS, Thatcher CD, Remillard RL, et al., eds. *Small Animal Clinical Nutrition, 4th Edition.* Topeka, KS: Mark Morris Institute, 213–260.

24. Kays RW, DeWan AA. 2004. Ecological impact of inside/outside house cats around a suburban nature preserve. *Animal Conservation* 7:1–11.

25. Muller G. 2006. The Social Role of Food and Behavioral Pathologies in the Dog. In: Pibot P, Biourge V, Elliot D, eds. *Encyclopedia of Canine Clnical Nutrition*. Europe: Diffo Print Italia, 452–461.

26. Horwitz D, Soulard Y, Junien-Castagna A. 2008. The Feeding Behavior of the Bat. In: Pibot P, Biourge V, Elliot D, eds. *Encyclopedia of Feline Clinical Nutrition*. Europe: Diffo Print Italia, 439–477.

27. Kirk CA, Debraekeleer J, Amstrong PJ. 2000. Normal Cats. In: Hand MS, Thatcher CD, Remillard RL, et al., eds. *Small Animal Clinical Nutrition. 4th Edition*. Topeka, KS: Mark Morris Institute, 291–347.

28. Buffington CA. 2009. Indoor Cat Initiative. Columbus: The Ohio State University College of Veterinary Medicine.

29. Burns KM. 2006. Managing overweight or obese pets. *Veterinary Technician* 27:385–389.

30. Moore A. 2004. *Healthy Dog: The Ultimate Fitness Guide for You and Your Dog*. Irvine: Bow Tie Press.

Nutritional Management of Obesity

Todd L. Towell, DVM, MS, DACVIM, and S. Dru Forrester, DVM, MS, DACVIM

Lose 30 pounds in 30 days! Fat is bad! Carbohydrates are bad! No need to count calories! Lose weight without exercising! These are all familiar claims made by a variety of manufacturers of weight loss products for people. In reality, weight loss requires an individual to consume fewer calories than they burn on a daily and sustained basis. But the "eat less and exercise more" message is not nearly as exciting as losing 30 pounds in 30 days or attributing weight gain to a specific nutrient. Indeed, the appeal of losing weight quickly is hard to resist.

But do weight-loss products, particularly dietary supplements, lighten anything but your wallet? Retail sales of weight loss supplements for humans exceed $1 billion despite lack of evidence of effectiveness for most products. Will avoiding specific nutrients prevent weight gain and increase weight loss? The retail sales of self help and weight loss publications in the United States exceeds $10 billion. It is often difficult for the average consumer to separate fact from fiction. Weak clinical and anecdotal or testimonial evidence is often used to support these types of claims.[1] This is true for both human and veterinary products. Application of the concepts of evidence-based medicine can assist veterinarians and health care team members sort fact from fiction. Before evaluating the evidence for weight loss claims it is important to have a general understanding of the basics of evidence-based decision making.

Practical Weight Management in Dogs and Cats, First Edition. Edited by Todd L. Towell.
© 2011 John Wiley and Sons, Inc. Published 2011 by John Wiley & Sons, Inc.

Evidence-based Veterinary Medicine

Evidence-based veterinary medicine (EBVM) is defined as the integration of the best research evidence, clinical expertise, available resources, and patient/client values. Best research evidence means clinically relevant research, especially from patient-centered clinical studies. Clinical expertise refers to the ability to use clinical skills and past experience to rapidly identify each patient's unique health status, establish a diagnosis, and determine the risks and benefits of potential interventions for that specific patient. Clinically relevant decisions also must take into account the resources (products, diagnostics tests or therapies) currently available. Patient/client values include unique preferences, concerns, and expectations each owner/patient brings to a clinical encounter and that must be integrated into clinical decisions to best serve the patient.

Integration of these four elements results in clinicians and owners forming a diagnostic and therapeutic alliance that optimizes clinical outcomes and quality of life (Figure 4.1). The intent is not to use current best evidence to replace clinical skills, judgment, or experience, but to provide another dimension to the decision-making process. Evidence-based veterinary medicine does not always lead to a definitive answer,

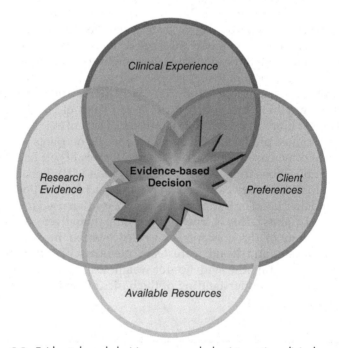

Figure 4.1. Evidence-based decisions are made by integrating clinical experience, client preferences, available resources, and best research evidence.

but it does provide a framework for making decisions and understanding the risk-benefit relationship of various therapeutic plans. Application of these principles can provide the foundation for the health care team to provide guidance to owners. To better understand EBVM, an understanding of the rules of evidence is necessary.

Rules of Evidence

The health care team should consider the quality of data supporting a recommendation to use (or not use) a specific treatment when prioritizing therapeutic recommendations. A classification scheme has been proposed for veterinary clinical nutrition and may be useful for establishing rules or dimensions of evidence for recommendations regarding weight management in pets.[2] Scientific evidence is the product of appropriately designed and carefully controlled research investigations. A single study does not constitute evidence; rather, it contributes to a body of knowledge that has been derived from multiple studies investigating the same area.

Traditional sources of evidence include textbooks, personal journal collections, conference proceedings, and clinical guidelines. However, much of this evidence is not based on appropriately conducted clinical studies in the target species. Many clinical interventions are used because the basic pathophysiologic rationale made sense, even though data documenting a positive effect on the clinical outcome are lacking. Sources regarded as strong evidence include randomized controlled clinical studies or systematic reviews of more than one study (i.e., meta-analysis). These are followed respectively by epidemiologic studies (cohort studies or case-control studies), models of disease, and case series. The hierarchy of evidence is based on the notion of causation and the need to control bias.

Evidence-based medicine guidelines for veterinary clinical nutrition have been outlined.[2] This scoring system recognizes that the quality of the evidence supporting a recommendation is an important consideration when making therapeutic decisions. Guidelines categorize the quality of evidence into the following grades: Grades I and II are the evidence with the highest quality, that is, grade I and II studies are most likely to predict results seen in clinical practice (Figure 4.2).

- Grade I: Evidence obtained from at least one properly designed, randomized, controlled study in the target species
- Grade II: Evidence obtained from at least one properly designed, randomized, controlled study in the target species but performed in a laboratory or research colony setting
- Grade III: Evidence obtained from appropriately controlled studies without randomization; evidence obtained from appropriately designed cohort or case-control studies, preferably from more than one center or research group; or dramatic results for uncontrolled

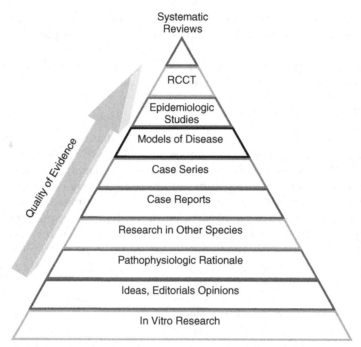

Figure 4.2. Grades of evidence. RCCT = Randomized controlled clinical trial.

studies (e.g., results for taurine supplementation in cats with cardio-myopathy), models of disease.

- Grade IV: Reports of expert committees, descriptive studies, case reports, and opinions of respected experts developed on the basis of their clinical experience. *In vitro* studies, extrapolations from other species.

Applying Evidence to a Specific Patient

The principles of EBVM do not preclude making clinical decisions based on Grade III or IV evidence if that is all that is available. However, the best application of EBVM occurs when decisions are based on a combination of the highest grade of evidence and clinical experience, client concerns, and available resources.

Even when data from clinical studies are available, several questions can be used to decide the applicability of evidence to nutritionally manage a specific patient. Were outcomes of the study clinically relevant? Are there differences between the animals in the study and my patient that may alter expected treatment response? Are there potential drug-nutrient interactions that may alter the expected treatment response? Are there differences in the nutrient contents of the food or supplements that may alter the expected treatment response? Is the food or supplement readily available and economically feasible? Is the nutritional intervention feasible in the owner's setting? What are the patient's likely benefits and risks from the various nutritional management options? How will the owner's values or patient's preferences influence the decision about nutritional management? Does the patient have other health conditions that substantially alter the potential benefits and risks of nutritional management?

Currently, veterinarians are taught to practice clinical medicine primarily on the basis of knowledge gained during their education and from continuing education programs, journals and textbooks, expert opinions, and their own experience of clinical success. These sources are usually relevant but often lack scientific scrutiny; frequently, these sources do not constitute the highest quality of evidence. In the future, veterinarians will increasingly need to understand the epidemiologic aspects of disease, apply clinical guidelines to specific patients, and discuss the risk-benefit probability with pet owners. Application of EBVM to veterinary medicine clearly offers a new approach for making clinical decisions and managing patient care. Adopting guidelines for veterinary clinical practice that include elements of EBVM and adapting them to each patient will likely improve patient outcomes.

These principles certainly apply to weight management in dogs and cats. Successful treatment and prevention of overweight and obese cats and dogs requires a multidimensional approach. The cornerstones of weight loss in any species are restriction of calorie intake (diet) and increase in calories expended (exercise). But what is the best way to restrict calorie intake? Are there nutrients or supplements that can enhance the success of weight loss programs? The following discussion examines these questions.

Nutraceuticals

Nutraceuticals (dietary supplements) can be described as a cross between food and pharmaceuticals. Veterinary nutraceuticals have been defined as nondrug substances that are produced in a purified or extracted form and administered orally to provide agents required for normal body structure and function with the intent of improving the health and well being of animals. Simply put, they are natural compounds that have health-promoting, disease-preventing, or medicinal properties that do not require a prescription.

In October 1994, the Dietary Supplement Health and Education Act (DSHEA) was signed into law by President Bill Clinton. Before this time, dietary supplements were subject to the same regulatory requirements as other foods. This new law, which amended the Federal Food, Drug, and Cosmetic Act, created a new regulatory framework for the safety and labeling of dietary supplements. Under DSHEA, a firm is responsible for determining that the dietary supplements it manufactures or distributes are safe and that any representations or claims made about them are substantiated by adequate evidence to show that they are not false or misleading. This means that dietary supplements do not need approval from the Food and Drug Administration (FDA) before they are marketed.

Except in the case of a new dietary ingredient, where pre-market review for safety data and other information is required by law, a firm does not have to provide the FDA with the evidence it relies on to substantiate safety or effectiveness before or after it markets its products. Under DSHEA, once the product is marketed, FDA has the responsibility for showing that a dietary supplement is "unsafe" before it can take action to restrict the product's use or removal from the marketplace. However, manufacturers and distributors of dietary supplements must record, investigate, and forward to the FDA any reports they receive of serious adverse events associated with the use of their products that are reported to them directly.

Key Point

Dietary supplements do not need approval from the FDA before they are marketed. The FDA must demonstrate a dietary supplement is unsafe before it takes action.

A variety of nutraceuticals or dietary supplements have been touted as aids for weight loss or management in veterinary patients. A recent review applied the aforementioned evidence-based guidelines to the data supporting the use of these supplements.[3] A summary of the reviewed products and supporting evidence is provided in Table 4.1. On the basis of this grading system, the best evidence exists for use of dietary l-carnitine supplementation in obese or overweight pets. More research-based evidence is needed to support routine recommendations of other nutraceuticals or dietary supplementation, such as pyruvate, amylase inhibitors, dehydroepiandrosterone (DHEA), conjugated linoleic acid (CLA), diacylglycerol, chromium, or vitamin A, for weight loss in pets.

Nutrigenomics: The Future of Functional Foods

Efforts to unravel the etiology of disease often have languished on the nature-vs.-nurture debate. Is it the genes you are born with or the environment you are exposed to that ultimately determines health or disease? Recent advances suggest that neither nature nor nurture alone

Table 4.1. Summary of evidence for use of nutraceuticals for weight loss in dogs and cats.

Supplement	Claim	Grade of evidence	Safety	Evidence supports use in dogs or cats
Pyruvate	Unknown	Grade II study in dogs: No effect		No
Omega-3 fatty acid	Regulate energy expenditure through mitochondrial uncoupling proteins	Grade II study in dogs		May be beneficial
Amylase inhibitors	Prevent digestion of complex carbohydrates	Grade IV in dogs and cats. Human studies: no effect		None available
Dehydroepiandrosterone (DHEA)	Induce thermogenic enzymes, increase resting heat production, impair fat synthesis, and promote lean tissue	Grade II study in dogs	Undesirable adverse effects associated with excessive amounts of sex hormones limit use	No
l-carnitine	Increases energy metabolism, helps burn fat while maintaining lean muscle mass, decreases the accumulation of fat in liver cells in cats.	Grade I and Grade II studies in dogs and cats		Yes
Conjugated linoleic acid (CLA)	Increases metabolic rate and energy expenditure, increases fatty acid oxidation, and reduces energy intake	Variable results, mostly abstracts	Possibly safe	May be beneficial for growing dogs, no clear evidence for adult dogs or cats
Dietary phytoestrogens	Moderate hyperglycemia and reduce body weight, hyperlipidemia, and hyperinsulinemia, particularly in gonadectomized animals	Grade II studies in dogs and cats	Longer term studies needed to assess safety	May be beneficial, more studies needed
Diacylglycerol	Alters fatty acid metabolism in the liver, lowers plasma triglyceride concentrations, decreases postprandial hyperlipidemia, increases energy expenditure, alters body composition	Grade II studies in dogs		May be beneficial, more studies needed
Chromium	Role in regulation of body composition is controversial, may increase lean body mass, decrease appetite, ± increase calories burned	Grade II studies in dogs and cats, no effect	Likely safe	More studies needed
Vitamin A	Inhibits leptin production, increases energy expenditure	Grade II studies indicate it may blunt weight gain		More studies needed

Adapted from Roudebush P, Schoenherr WD, Delaney SJ. 2008. An evidence-based review of the use of nutraceuticals and dietary supplementation for the management of obese and overweight pets. *J Am Vet Med Assoc* 232:1646–1655.

can explain the molecular processes that ultimately govern health. In most cases, the presence of a particular gene or mutation merely indicates a predisposition to a particular disease process. Whether that genetic potential will manifest as a disease depends on elaborate interactions between the genome and environmental factors.

Prior to the advent of genomic technologies, changes in gene expression attributed to diet were thought to be mediated through endocrine or neural pathways. However, research has shown that macronutrients, micronutrients, and their metabolites can directly regulate gene expression. Indeed, diet is arguably one of the most important environmental factors influencing health and disease. Although genes are critical for determining predilections, nutrition modifies the extent to which different genes are expressed and thereby modulates whether individuals fully express the promise established by their genetic background. Simply put, genes load the gun but environment pulls the trigger.

Key Point

Diet is one of the most important environmental factors influencing health and disease.

Associations between diet and disease have long been recognized through epidemiological studies. New genomic technologies, the so-called "-omics tools," are now elucidating the basis of these associations. These technologies monitor the activity of multiple genes simultaneously at the level of RNA by transcriptomics, the level of the proteins by proteomics, and ultimately the level of metabolites by metabolomics. All of these "-omics tools" have been used to study in detail the molecular responses to nutrients and the early stages of disease in common diet-related conditions.

Key Point

Nutrigenomics is the study of the effect of nutrients on gene expression, proteins, and metabolites.

Nutrigenetics

The term nutrigenetics is used to describe the effect of genotype on nutrient absorption, metabolism, transport, and excretion. An animal's response to a specific nutrient, for example, may depend on the DNA sequence of the genes and consequent structures of the proteins involved with its absorption and metabolism. While DNA sequences may be altered in several ways, the simplest change is known as a single nucleotide polymorphism (SNP), in which one nucleotide base is replaced with another. Single nucleotide polymorphisms may be thought of as variations in a recipe. If each gene is a recipe for a specific protein that performs a given biological function, then the nucleotides may be likened to the ingredients. As in many recipes, the effects of substituting one ingredient for another may be severe, mild, or undetectable. SNPs that change the recipe significantly, resulting in a different quantity or type of protein, may ultimately alter an animal's response to diet or susceptibility to disease.

One recent example of the application of nutrigenetics to canine genetic diseases involves the study of inherited copper toxicosis of Bedlington Terriers (CTBT). CTBT is a copper-associated hepatopathy caused by an autosomal recessive genetic defect of copper metabolism. Although this disease has been studied for decades, it has only been recently found to be caused by a mutation in the MURR1 gene, with several genetic variants (i.e., SNPs) associated with the disease.[4] An MURR1 mutation results in defective copper metabolism, allowing copper to accumulate in hepatic tissue. Historically, the best method for diagnosis was measuring hepatic copper concentrations at 1 year of age. However, hepatic copper concentrations already may be dangerously high by that time. Additionally, because hepatic copper concentrations are not elevated in animals carrying only one mutated allele, this measurement could not identify carriers of the disease. Currently a genetic test enables screening for MURR1 mutations, identifying affected animals and carriers of the mutation. Genetic testing may be performed soon after birth, allowing the owner and veterinarian to modify the diet accordingly.

Nutrigenomics

Contrary to nutrigenetics, nutrigenomics analyzes the effects of nutrients on the gene expression, proteins, and metabolites. Nutrients can be thought of as dietary signals detected by cellular sensor systems that influence gene expression and subsequently protein and metabolite production. Recurring patterns of gene expression, protein, and metabolite production in response to particular nutrients or foods can be viewed as dietary signatures. Nutrigenomics studies these signatures to understand how nutrition influences health and disease (Figure 4.3).

One potential outcome from nutrigenomics research is a more rational approach to food formulation. Based on a more comprehensive understanding of the effects of diet on health, foods can be designed to modify expression profiles in affected animals to more closely reflect a healthy state. Traditionally, the role of nutrition in the management of diseases has focused on correcting deficiencies or avoiding excesses of

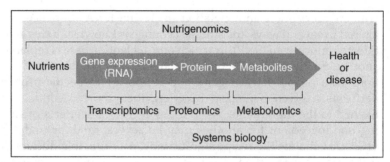

Figure 4.3. A schematic overview of the relationships between nutrigenomics, transcriptomics, proteomics, metabolomics, and systems biology. Used with permission: Al-Murrani S, Thatcher CD, Hand MS. 2010. Nutrigenomics and Nutrigenetics: Nutritional Genomics in Health and Disease. In: Hand MS, Thatcher CD, Remillard RL, et al., eds. *Small Animal Clinical Nutrition,* 5th ed. Topeka, KS: Mark Morris Institute, 44.

specific nutrients. As such, nutrition has been relegated to a supportive therapy role similar to fluid therapy, not as a primary means of ameliorating diseases. The recent advances in nutrigenomics have led to a better understanding of how nutrients can directly modulate pathophysiological processes, elevating nutrition to a primary means of both preventing and managing diseases.[5]

Nutrigenomics and Obesity

Nutrigenomic studies have enabled scientists to identify consistent differences in gene expression between lean and obese individuals. The gene expression of obese adipocytes showed a down-regulation of PPAR-gamma, uncoupling protein-2, carnitine O-palmitoyltransferase 1 A, and acyl-CoA synthetase. When functioning properly, these genes are important in the beta-oxidation of fatty acids. The down-regulation of these genes may explain why obese animals are fat storing instead of fat burning (Figure 4.4).

Employing the results of nutrigenomic research allows for an innovative approach to the formulation of a therapeutic food for weight loss. Using these principles, the nutrient profile is selected based on an understanding of how specific nutrients alter gene expression. For the obese dog, the goal is to alter gene expression to more closely resemble that of a lean individual (fat burner rather than fat storer).

A recent study evaluated the effects of weight loss on the gene expression profiles of obese dogs.[6] These obese dogs (greater than 35% body fat by DEXA) were fed a dry, low-fat, fiber-enhanced therapeutic food (Hill's® Prescription Diet® r/d® Canine dry; 33.2% crude protein, 8.7% crude fat, and 26.7% total dietary fiber on dry matter basis) for

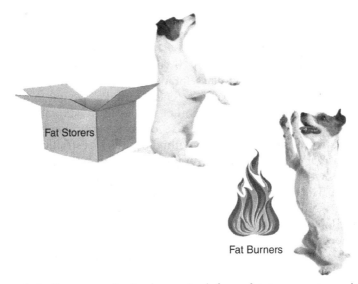

Figure 4.4. Gene expression in obese animals favors fat storage, compared to lean individuals, in which gene expression favors fat burning. Images from Fotolia.com.

four months. On average, dogs lost 2.8 ± 0.8 kg body fat (41.2% of initial fat mass) in four months, which is neither unusual nor remarkable.

What is remarkable is the observed shift from obese to a lean gene expression profile in these dogs. Of the genes identified, there was a down-regulation of genes associated with fat accumulation (i.e., leptin and IGF-1) once the dogs lost weight. This data suggests that obese dogs fed the weight loss food had a shift in metabolism to a lean genomic profile. Dogs were both phenotypically and metabolically lean.

Interestingly, weight loss alone does not alter gene expression. In an identical study, obese dogs (greater than 35% body fat by DEXA) were fed a dry, low-fiber, high-protein, moderate fat therapeutic food (47.5% crude protein, 27.1% crude fat, and 6.2% total dietary fiber on dry matter basis) for four months. On average, dogs lost 3 ± 0.4 kg body fat (44.9% of initial fat mass) in four months. These dogs were phenotypically lean; however, gene expression was not altered once these dogs reached ideal weight. Changes in gene expression occur as a result of foods formulated with specific nutrient profiles and weight loss working together.

Key Point

Changes in gene expression occur as a result of foods formulated with specific nutrient profiles and weight loss working together.

Therapeutic Weight Loss Foods

Therapeutic weight loss foods have been used in dogs for more than 50 years and cats for more than 20 years.[7] There are several benefits of using this specific food class for weight loss. Unhealthy weight gain develops secondary to excessive energy intake. Weight loss is induced by calorie restriction, which can be achieved by starvation, reduction of intake of current food, or use of therapeutic weight loss foods. Starvation is an unacceptable method of calorie restriction in obese cats because of the risk of hepatic lipidosis. In dogs, starvation can be effective; however, 10% to 25% of the resulting weight loss comes from lean tissue.[8] The loss of lean body mass reduces maintenance energy requirement, which ultimately sabotages the weight management program. Needless to say, starvation diets are generally unsustainable for most owners.

Restricting the amount of the pet's current food may seem like a reasonable approach to many owners. However, this strategy is generally neither effective nor ideal. Maintenance type pet foods are nutritionally balanced based on their energy density. For pets to receive the recommended amounts of nutrients (e.g., protein, essential fatty acids, vitamins, minerals) they must consume amounts of the food consistent with the expected calorie intake. When calorie intake is reduced, intake of all nutrients, not just energy, is restricted. If the amount of maintenance food is markedly decreased, deficiencies in some beneficial nutrients may occur. Additionally, because maintenance foods are not designed to enhance satiety, this method will likely result in increased begging behavior and failure of the weight loss program. It is important that the food chosen for calorie restriction have an increased nutrient/calorie ratio to avoid restriction of essential nutrients, is formulated to enhance satiety, and has evidence supporting its efficacy in weight loss programs. Therapeutic weight loss foods are specifically formulated to address these needs.

Key Points

Therapeutic weight loss foods help pets keep the muscle and lose the fat.

The goal of any weight loss program is reduction of body fat while preserving lean body mass. Traditional therapeutic weight loss foods for dogs and cats rely on a low-fat, high-fiber composition to accomplish this goal. This nutrient profile helps reduce caloric intake, decrease body weight, and maintain satiety and lean body mass. In cats, a newer concept involves using therapeutic weight loss foods with a high-protein, low-carbohydrate composition. This nutrient profile also results in a decrease body weight and reduced loss of lean body mass. An evidence-based review of the available research evaluating various commercial therapeutic weight foods for weight management in both species can be found in the literature.[7]

Canine Therapeutic Weight Loss Foods

Little is known about the relative efficacy of commercially available weight loss products in pet dogs in the home setting, although there is a growing body of evidence. Traditionally, clinical studies for weight management have been conducted in laboratory animals. In such studies, weight loss, changes in body composition (body fat and lean body mass), and metabolic changes (blood lipid concentrations, liver enzyme activity, and glucose tolerance) have been evaluated. Dogs participating in laboratory studies routinely lose weight. Anecdotally, clinical experience with therapeutic foods may not be as reliable. One notable difference between weight loss studies in laboratory dogs and client-owned dogs is compliance. In the laboratory setting, adherence to the prescribed dose of food is 100%; sadly, this is not always true in the home setting. The reasons for lack of compliance by owners are numerous. However, two issues may play key roles in preventing successful weight loss in the home environment: begging behavior and rate of weight loss.

Key Point

Keys to Success: Minimize begging, maximize rate of weight loss.

Satiety

In the home setting, satiety is particularly important to the success of a weight management program. When dogs do not feel full, they beg. Most owners provide additional calories in the form of treats or additional food in response to begging behavior. Increased fiber content of therapeutic weight loss foods is one strategy for minimizing begging. Whether increased dietary fiber results in increased satiety or fullness is difficult to prove in people and even more so in dogs because it is a subjective feeling often measured by lack of desire to eat. Despite this challenge, increased dietary fiber intake has been associated with decreased food intake for up to eight hours in people.[9,10]

Results of studies in dogs are variable; some show no effect on caloric intake whereas others document a benefit. In one study, increased fiber did not produce any difference in satiety.[11] However, in this study dogs were fed 40% of calories for maintenance. This severe calorie restriction may have overshadowed any effect of fiber between groups. In a study designed to assess the effect of fiber on satiety in dogs offered maintenance calories, dogs consuming high-fiber food voluntarily ate significantly less food than dogs in the lower fiber group.[12]

Key Point

High-fiber foods decrease snacking in dogs.

Rate of Weight Loss

The primary predictor of initial and long-term success of weight management programs in people is the rate of weight loss.[13] A recent study has documented both short- and long-term advantages to fast initial weight loss in people. Participants who lost weight rapidly lost more weight, kept it off longer, and were not more susceptible to weight regain than those who lost weight gradually.[14] Although similar studies have not been conducted in client-owned dogs, it is reasonable to predict that owners will be more prone to continue a weight loss program if they see rapid results in their dogs.

Compared to maintenance foods, therapeutic weight loss foods are designed to enhance satiety and ensure consistent weight loss.[15–19] The ideal proportion of protein and fiber to achieve rapid and consistent weight loss is not known. Products with a wide range of protein (24% to 47% on a dry matter basis) and fiber (3% to 39% total daily fiber on a dry matter basis) contents have been shown to be effective. Based on published studies, products with lower fat and higher fiber result in greater, more rapid loss of body fat compared to higher fat, lower fiber foods.[17,19,20] Because owners are more likely to continue a weight management program if they see results, these lower fat/higher fiber foods may be the best choice.

Dietary Protein

Dietary protein has several key effects that benefit weight loss. To prevent loss of lean body mass, dogs undergoing weight loss require increased protein. However, it is not simply the quantity of protein that is important in protecting against the loss of lean body mass, but also the quality of protein.[21] Protein quality depends on the amino acids that make up the protein. Once ingested, proteins are broken down into their constituent amino acids. Each necessary amino acid must be available in adequate amounts for the amino acids to be used for protein synthesis. The amino acid that is in the shortest supply is referred to as the first limiting amino acid. Using foods formulated to ensure adequate levels of necessary amino acids in overweight dogs has shown promising results in the maintenance of lean body mass during weight loss.

One study compared two foods with similar protein and fiber content: 33.5% dry matter (DM) protein and about 10.5% DM crude fiber. The foods differed in that the experimental food contained increased soluble fiber and had an optimized amino acid ratio with a higher lysine-to-calorie content. Compared to dogs fed the control food, dogs fed the experimental food lost significantly more body weight (-2.1 kg vs. -1.3 kg, respectively) and actually gained rather than lost lean body mass during weight loss (approximately +0.3 kg vs. –1.1 kg, respectively).[21] Unfortunately, the lysine content of a food is not reflected by crude protein content. Although not perfect, the total amount of lysine in dog foods for weight management is somewhat indicative of how "perfect" the food's protein content is. Lysine content of foods should be available from the manufacturer.

> ## Key Point
>
> Quality of protein may be more important than quantity. Lysine content is a measure of the quality of protein..

Carbohydrates

Carbohydrates are an often maligned nutrient, particularly in the lay press with regard to human weight control. There are three main categories of carbohydrates: simple sugars, complex carbohydrates, and dietary fiber. The importance of dietary fiber in weight loss has been discussed. The remaining categories, simple sugars and complex carbohydrates (grain sources), are the focus of many weight loss programs for humans because of their effects on glycemic index. Originally developed as a tool to help people with diabetes manage blood sugar control, the glycemic index has found its way into the mainstream weight loss market. The glycemic index is the basis for many popular diet plans, such as South Beach, The Zone, Sugar Busters, Glucose Revolution, and Ending the Food Fight.

In humans, the glycemic index (GI) measures how much a 50-gram portion of carbohydrate raises a person's blood-sugar levels compared with a control (white bread or pure glucose). In both people and pets, virtually all carbohydrates except fiber are digested into glucose and cause a temporary rise in blood glucose levels, called the glycemic response. This response is affected by many factors, including the quantity of food, the amount and type of carbohydrate, the cooking method, and the degree of processing, to name a few. Despite the proliferation of diets and books based on the glycemic index, some researchers and experts are unconvinced that this number truly holds value in everyday life, where food is eaten as part of a mixed meal.

A study designed to test the accuracy of glycemic index tables to predict the glycemic index of a variety of typical breakfast meals concluded that the table values for glycemic index did not predict the measured glycemic index.[22] Interestingly, these researchers found that the combined content of fat and protein in a meal, as well as total energy, were stronger predictors of glycemic index than the carbohydrate content alone. These findings confirm that interactions of complex meals play an important role in the absorption and metabolism of individual nutrients.

Compared to humans, there is relatively little information about glycemic index in dogs. However, consumption of different sugars and carbohydrate sources has been shown to alter postprandial glucose levels and insulin secretory patterns in dogs.[23-25] Consequently, it has been suggested that foods producing low glycemic responses be fed to diabetic and obese dogs, as well as for prevention of these conditions.

In a study that evaluated the effects of feeding five different carbohydrate sources (corn, wheat, barley, rice, and sorghum) on glucose and insulin responses in dogs, rice had the highest postprandial glycemic response (i.e., increased postprandial glucose and insulin response).[23] Barley, corn, and sorghum were the best carbohydrate sources for dogs with impaired glucose control (i.e., diabetes and obesity) because of their low-insulinogenic responses.[23] For this reason it is important to evaluate the carbohydrate sources of weight management foods. Based on these findings, it is best to avoid foods based primarily on rice when selecting weight-loss foods. By convention, ingredients are listed in descending order of volume by weight on a dog food product's ingredient label. Therefore, the earlier rice is listed on the ingredient label, the more rice the product contains. Arbitrarily, rice should not be one of the first three or four non-water ingredients on a weight-loss or weight-control food's label.

Selecting a Food
Prescribing a therapeutic weight loss food is preferable to restricting the amount of maintenance foods for dogs in a weight loss program. Therapeutic weight loss foods are formulated to ensure that restricting calories does not mean restriction of other important nutrients. The specific product that is best for each pet may vary; however, research supports the use of lower fat, higher fiber foods to increase satiety and decrease begging behavior in dogs. New information indicates that it is possible to alter gene expression in overweight dogs with foods formulated based on nutrigenomic studies. Finally, the quality of protein in canine weight loss foods appears to be more important than the quantity.

Feline Therapeutic Weight Loss Foods

A variety of commercially available therapeutic weight loss foods for cats have been evaluated by clinical studies. These studies in obese cats have been conducted with low-fat, low-fiber dry food; low-fat, high-fiber moist and dry foods; high-fat, low-carbohydrate, moderate-fiber moist and dry foods; and high-protein, low-fat, moderate-fiber dry food.[26] All published studies document significant decreases in weight and body fat and no significant loss in lean body mass when the commercial therapeutic foods were fed to obese cats. Diet-induced weight loss also appears to improve glucose tolerance, minimize oxidative damage to tissues, and improve the inflammatory status in obese cats.[27,28]

Recently the use of low-carb foods for weight loss in cats has gained popularity, similar to the resurgence of this approach to human weight loss programs. The first low-carbohydrate diet for people was used in the 1860s.[29] Contemporary versions of this theme include the Atkins and South Beach diet programs. Although these diets emphasize lowering carbohydrate intake, both rely on a multifaceted approach including decreasing fat intake, use of lower glycemic index carbohydrate sources, and to some extent increasing dietary fiber. The primary effect of these diet recommendations for humans is to lower the consumption of calories as refined carbohydrates and fructose (sugar).

This is important for human health, as recent studies support a direct link between consumption of refined carbohydrates and fructose and metabolic syndrome. A study designed to examine the nutrient consumption of the typical diet in the United States between 1909 and 1997 found a significant correlation in the prevalence of diabetes with fat, carbohydrate, corn syrup, and total energy intake.[30] Strikingly, when total energy intake was accounted for, corn syrup was positively associated with type 2 diabetes, whereas protein and fat were not.

High-fructose corn syrup is commonly found in soft drinks, juice beverages, and many convenient prepackaged foods such as baked goods. In fact, in the United States consumption of fructose as a component of high-fructose corn syrup has increased an astounding 1,000% between 1970 and 1990.[31] In 1970 the average person consumed a mere 0.5 lbs/year. By 1997 this figure was estimated at an shocking 62.4 lbs/year.[32] By encouraging people to minimize the consumption of prepackaged, prepared foods in favor of fresh vegetables and fruits, the consumption of refined carbohydrates (sugars) and fructose is minimized.

It is interesting to note that despite the media blitz touting the benefits of low-carbohydrate diets in people, results of clinical studies show little difference in the long term between low-carbohydrate and traditional low-fat diets. Early studies suggested that more early weight loss occurs with low-carbohydrate diets than with low-fat diets. However, in a study specifically designed to compare the long-term results of low-carbohydrate and low-fat diets, after two years, participants lost an average of 7 kg or 7% of body weight, and no differences between the two groups were found.[33]

Regardless, the popularity of these strategies for humans has caused them to spill over to other species. While these strategies may be important means of improving human health, it is not always appropriate to extrapolate these findings to other species. In cats, the use of metabolic controls foods (low-carb) is an alternative to calorie control foods for weight loss. The basic premise of the metabolic approach is to shift energy metabolism from energy storage to energy use. For safe weight loss in cats, clinical trials have shown the efficacy of metabolic control foods to be equivalent to tradition low-calorie (higher fiber) foods. Nonetheless, a variety of myths and misconceptions regarding carbohydrates and cats still abound. The following discussion summarizes the current information on this topic.

Cats and Carbohydrates: What Do We Really Know?

The role of carbohydrates (and dry food) in the pathogenesis of feline diseases such as obesity and diabetes mellitus currently is a topic of considerable discussion and debate.[34-38] Cats are carnivores that have adapted to foods higher in protein and lower in carbohydrates, compared with other species (e.g., dogs).[38,39] It has been suggested or stated that increased consumption of carbohydrates in dry commercial pet foods is the cause for increased occurrence of feline diseases and that feeding low-carbohydrate foods may be indicated to prevent or manage these conditions.[35,36,39-43] The primary purpose of this section is to summarize what is currently known about the role of carbohydrates (and dry food) in the pathogenesis of obesity and diabetes mellitus in cats and review evidence that supports feeding low-carbohydrate foods to cats with diabetes mellitus or obesity.

Are Cats Capable of Digesting and Using Carbohydrates?

The natural prey of cats includes small rodents, which are estimated to contain around 55% protein, 45% fat, and little carbohydrate (1% to 2%) on a dry matter basis (Figure 4.5).[38,44] The average carbohydrate content (% dry matter; DM) of dry grocery brand cat foods is 44%, whereas moist grocery brand cat foods contain approximately 10% carbohydrates.[45] Because of physiologic differences in cats (e.g., low hepatic glucokinase activity, decreased activities of intestinal and pancreatic amylase) and results of some studies evaluating carbohydrate digestion, it has been suggested that cats cannot efficiently use carbohydrates and that carbohydrates decrease protein digestibility.[38,46,47] These studies included simple sugars (e.g., glucose) and raw carbohydrates, and most commercial pet foods contain complex carbohydrates that are pro-

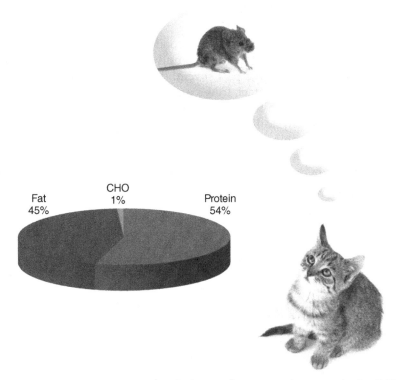

Figure 4.5. Nutrient content of typical prey of cats on a dry matter basis. CHO = carbohydrate. Courtesy Hill's Pet Nutrition, Inc.

cessed.[46,47] When appropriately processed carbohydrates (ground and cooked) are fed to cats, they are highly digestible (greater than 90%) and are not associated with clinically important decreases in protein digestibility.[46,48–50]

Although a dietary requirement does not exist for carbohydrates in cats (or dogs or people), carbohydrates are an excellent source of energy. Most cells use glucose as their primary source of energy. When carbohydrates are provided in the diet, they serve as a readily available source for production of glucose. In their absence, amino acids are diverted from protein synthesis to produce glucose (i.e., gluconeogenesis). When energy needs are high (e.g., growth, gestation, lactation), carbohydrates become conditionally essential; therefore, foods for pets with high-energy demands (e.g., lactating queens) usually contain increased carbohydrates. In addition, carbohydrates provide structural integrity for dry food; starch works like a cement to hold kibble together and prevent crumbling during the manufacturing process.

Lifestyle and Management Factors That Affect the Health of Cats Today

When evaluating the role of dry food (and carbohydrates) in feline diseases, it is important to consider all changes that have occurred in the lives of cats over the past several decades (Table 4.2).

In contrast to the intact, free-roaming, and "working" cat of the past, most cats today are family pets that live indoors and are spayed or neutered, less physically active, and are fed dry food. It is possible that all or some combination of these factors have affected the occurrence of feline diseases, particularly obesity. In addition, many of the risk factors for being overweight or obese also are factors associated with diabetes mellitus (Table 4.3).

Table 4.2. Changes in cats' lives over the past several decades.

	Past	Present
Environment	Outside	Indoors
Lifestyle	Free roaming	Sedentary, physically inactive
Reproductive status	Intact	Spayed/neutered
Food source/type	Prey, table scraps	Commercial food (most often dry)
Food acquisition	Hunting	Waiting for bowl to be filled
Function	Reproduction	Family pet

Table 4.3. Risk factors for feline diseases.

	Obesity/ overweight	Diabetes mellitus
Age	Middle aged	Increasing age
Gender	Male	Male
Reproductive status	Neutered	Neutered
Breed	Several	Burmese
Physical activity	Decreased	Decreased
Environment	Indoors	Indoors
Body condition (% body fat)	Increased	Increased

Information compiled from: McCann TM, Simpson KE, Shaw DJ, et al. 2007. Feline diabetes mellitus in the UK: The prevalence within an insured cat population and a questionnaire-based putative risk factor analysis. J Feline Med Surg 9:289–299.

Panciera DL, Thomas CB, Eicker SW, et al. 1990. Epizootiologic patterns of diabetes mellitus in cats: 333 cases (1980–1986). J Am Vet Med Assoc 197:1504–1508.

Prahl A, Guptill L, Glickman NW, et al. 2007. Time trends and risk factors for diabetes mellitus in cats presented to veterinary teaching hospitals. J Feline Med Surg 9:351–358.

Slingerland LI, Fazilova VV, Plantinga EA, et al. 2009. Indoor confinement and physical inactivity rather than the proportion of dry food are risk factors in the development of feline type 2 diabetes mellitus. Vet J 179:247–253.

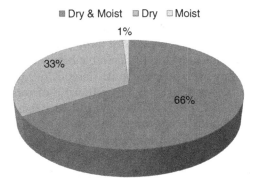

Figure 4.6. Feeding habits of 802 cat owners surveyed in 2002. The overwhelming majority (99%) responded that they fed either a mixture of moist and dry food or dry food alone, whereas only 1% fed moist food only. Source: Hill's Pet Nutrition Inc. Habits and Practices Study, 2002.

Table 4.4. How owners feed their cats (dry vs. moist food).

Frequency	Dry food	Moist food
Less than once daily	2%	18%
Once daily	22%	43%
Twice daily	19%	30%
Bowl is always full	51%	3%

Data collected from survey of 820 cat owners. Hill's Pet Nutrition Inc. Habits and Practices Study, 2002.

Feeding Practices

Most cat owners prefer to feed dry food, probably for reasons related to convenience (ease of food preparation, storage, and delivery) and cost (dry food is less expensive) (Figure 4.6).[51] Of cat owners that feed dry food, more than half keep the bowl full at all times, whereas people who feed moist (e.g., canned) food are more likely to provide their cats with one or two meals daily (Table 4.4). One study identified dry food as a risk factor for obesity.[52] However, several more recent studies have confirmed that free-choice feeding (whether canned or dry food) is associated with excessive caloric intake and increased body weight and fat in spayed and neutered cats.[50,53–63] Neutered cats eating a dry weight management food free choice became overweight; however, when they were fed a controlled amount of the same food, they lost weight successfully.[58]. Making food available at all times facilitates excessive caloric intake, which contributes to obesity. Because of feeding habits of cat owners, this is more likely to occur with dry food.

Spaying/Neutering

Most cats today, especially those that live indoors, are spayed or neutered. There are obvious benefits of these procedures including population control and decreasing undesirable behaviors (e.g., urine spraying or marking); however, there are nutritional consequences. Documented changes that occur after spaying/neutering of cats include decreased metabolic rate and physical activity and increased food intake, body weight, body condition score, and amount of body fat.[50,53–63–65] Metabolic changes are observed within days to weeks after spaying or neutering. In one study, caloric intake increased by 25% within four weeks of gonadectomy and by 50% within three months.[53] These changes appear to occur regardless of whether spaying or neutering is done at an early age (7 weeks) or later (7 months).[66]

Key Point

After neutering, caloric intake increased by 25% at one month and by 50% at three months.

The Role of Increased Carbohydrate (or Dry Food) Intake as a Cause of Diabetes Mellitus or Obesity in Cats

Several authors have stated that high-carbohydrate foods either cause or may be a factor in development of diabetes mellitus and/or obesity in cats.[35,36,39,40,42,43,67,68] The proposed pathogenesis is that carbohydrate consumption causes hyperglycemia, which stimulates insulin release and over time leads to pancreatic β-cell exhaustion and diabetes mellitus. There are many findings that do not support this theory, however. Below is a brief summary of the main points from studies that have evaluated the potential role of dietary carbohydrates in the pathogenesis of diabetes mellitus and obesity in cats.[47,48,50,53,58,69–76]

- Whereas consumption of simple sugars (e.g., glucose) resulted in increased blood glucose concentrations in healthy cats, cooked maize starch (a complex carbohydrate) did not.[47] Most commercial cat foods contain complex carbohydrates and not simple sugars; therefore, it seems unlikely that cats eating commercial dry foods would develop hyperglycemia.[34,37,77]
- Feeding a variety of commercial dry and canned cat foods to healthy and diabetic cats was not associated with a significant change in blood glucose concentration.[74]
- Compared with fasting values, no significant difference occurred in postprandial serum glucose concentrations when cats were fed two

dry commercial foods with 37% or 42% carbohydrates DM.[75] There was a significant decrease in serum glucose when cats were fed a dry food with 16% carbohydrates and 52% protein DM; however, serum insulin concentration increased significantly. The food containing the highest amount of carbohydrates (42% DM) was associated with the lowest serum insulin concentration.

- The feline pancreas appears more responsive to amino acids than glucose; therefore, dietary protein would be expected to stimulate pancreatic insulin secretion in cats.[78–80]
- In a study of healthy cats, feeding different carbohydrate sources had minimal impact on glucose and insulin responses.[48] Compared with the baseline, only the food with corn stimulated an increase in glucose response and these values were within the range considered normal for cats (mean plasma glucose concentration after eating was 79 mg/dl [4.39 mmol/L] and the highest plasma glucose concentration was 93 mg/dl [5.16 mmol/L]).
- Results of a preliminary study revealed that feeding a high-protein food (46% calories from protein) to healthy cats was associated with lower postprandial glucose concentrations compared with high-carbohydrate (47% calories from carbohydrates) or high-fat (47% calories from fat) foods.[70]
- In a different preliminary study, healthy cats fed a low-protein (28% of calories), low-fat (28% of calories), or low-carbohydrate (3% of calories) food had no differences in results of glucose tolerance testing.[76] Insulin concentration tended to be higher for the low-carbohydrate food (which contained the highest protein).
- In another preliminary study of healthy cats, feeding a high-protein (58% DM)/low-carbohydrate (8% DM) food was associated with mixed results compared with a low-protein (33% DM)/high-carbohydrate (33% DM) food.[71] There was no difference between groups in glucose concentrations after intravenous glucose challenge or food, and no difference in insulin concentrations after intravenous glucose. However, insulin was significantly greater after eating the low-protein/high-carbohydrate food.
- Healthy cats eating a high-fat food (with 13% carbohydrates DM) had significantly higher plasma glucose concentrations during glucose tolerance testing compared with cats eating a high-carbohydrate (40% DM)/low-fat food.[50] The authors concluded that a long-term study was needed to determine whether the amount of dietary fat, rather than dietary carbohydrate, might contribute to development of diabetes mellitus in cats.
- Regardless of dietary protein or carbohydrate content, obesity led to severe insulin resistance in a study of obese cats, and weight loss normalized insulin sensitivity.[72]
- In an epidemiological study, indoor confinement and low physical activity were identified as risk factors for diabetes mellitus; however, amount of dry food was not.[81]

- Effects of weight gain and feeding different amounts of carbohydrate (4%, 27%, 45%, or 56% carbohydrate, DM) and fat were evaluated in a study of healthy cats that were fed dry food free choice before and after neutering.[53] High dietary carbohydrate, relative to high fat, did not induce weight gain or increased plasma glucose and insulin concentrations in sexually intact cats. Gonadectomy stimulated food intake to the degree that undesired gains in body weight and fat occurred. The authors concluded that weight gain induced by high dietary fat and gonadectomy are probably more important to consider in the long-term health of cats than dietary carbohydrate content.

The majority of published evidence does not support a direct cause-and-effect relationship between increased carbohydrate or dry food intake and diabetes mellitus or obesity in cats.[34,37] It seems likely that a combination of factors plays a role and that increased dietary carbohydrates may be an indirect factor due to free-choice feeding of dry food (which is typically high in carbohydrates) and subsequent obesity, which is associated with insulin resistance (Figure 4.7). In other words, it's the calories, not the carbohydrates, that are more likely a nutritional cause for the epidemic of obesity and increased risk for diabetes mellitus in cats.

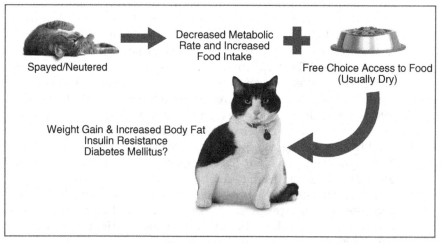

Figure 4.7. Spaying/neutering of cats is associated with decreased metabolic rate (decreased energy requirements), increased food intake, and decreased physical activity, which leads to obesity unless food intake is decreased. Most cats are fed dry food that often is available at all times; this further increases the likelihood of becoming overweight or obese. Increased body fat is associated with insulin resistance in cats, which could lead to development of diabetes mellitus. Used with permission from Dr. S. Dru Forrester.

Amount of Carbohydrates or Protein That Should be Fed to Cats with Diabetes Mellitus and/or Obesity

Some clinicians strongly caution that foods for diabetic cats must contain less than 7% carbohydrates (DM), and high-fiber foods are not appropriate. Published evidence does not support this recommendation, however. In addition, there is currently debate about the effect of different types of insulin on diabetic remission in cats.[40,82–84] A variety of insulin products were used in studies evaluating low-carbohydrate foods in diabetic cats, and this could have impacted treatment success regardless of diet.[85–88]

The goals for nutritional management of diabetic cats are to achieve/maintain ideal body weight and improve glycemic control, including discontinuation of insulin therapy. This has been accomplished by feeding a low-carbohydrate food or a low-fat/high-fiber food.[85,89] Feeding increased fiber, which may delay or decrease carbohydrate absorption from the gastrointestinal tract, has been associated with improved glycemic control in cats with diabetes mellitus.[85,90] In one study of diabetic cats managed with a high-fiber food for four months, 41% experienced remission (i.e., no longer needed insulin).[85] In the same study, feeding a low-carbohydrate/high-protein kitten food was associated with a significantly higher remission rate (68%). Studies of the effects of low-carbohydrate foods in diabetic cats reveal that a range of dietary carbohydrates (5% to 26% of calories) have been associated with diabetic remission in 17% to 68% of cats (Table 4.5).[85–88,91]

The highest remission rates occurred when cats were fed moist kitten foods with moderate amounts of protein (34% or 37% of calories) and 5% or 12% calories as carbohydrates.[85,87] The lowest remission rates occurred when cats were fed high-protein foods (46% to 50% of calories).[86,88,91] In two studies, cats fed dry and/or moist high-protein foods gained weight, most likely because dry food was offered free choice.[88,91] It is possible that weight gain, often associated with insulin resistance, resulted in lower remission rates. In another study evaluating a low-carbohydrate food, the best response was observed in obese cats, whereas cats with lower initial body fat continued to require insulin therapy to control clinical signs.[87] Based on these findings, it seems reasonable to conclude that weight loss alone may result in diabetic remission in overweight cats regardless of dietary nutrient intake (i.e., it's the calories, not the carbohydrates).

Key Point

It is calories, not the carbohydrates, that increase the risk of obesity and diabetes mellitus.

Table 4.5. Nutrient content of foods associated with remission in cats with diabetes mellitus.

Study food	Carb (% DM)	Carb (g/100kcal)	Carb (% ME)	Protein (% ME)	Crude fiber (g/100kcal)	Remission rate (%)	References
Purina Veterinary Diets DM, Dietetic Formula (can and dry)	NR	2.6–3.3	NR	12.5–13.9 (g/100kcal)	0.33–0.56	17	91
Purina Veterinary Diets DM, Dietetic Formula (can and dry)	8.1–15	1.7–3.4	6.6–13	46–50	0.3–0.8	31	88
Purina Veterinary Diets DM, Dietetic Formula (can)	8.1	1.7	6.6	46	0.8	33	86
Hill's® Prescription Diet® w/d® Feline (can)	NR	7.6	26	40	3.1	41	85
Hill's® Science Diet® Feline Growth (can)	6.9	1.3	5	34	0.1	63	87
Hill's® Science Diet® Feline Growth (can)	NR	3.5	12	37	0.1	68	85

Carb = carbohydrate, % DM = % dry matter, ME = metabolizable energy (calories), NR = not reported

As with diabetic cats, nutritional management of overweight or obese cats most often involves feeding either a low-fat/high-fiber food or a low-carbohydrate/high-protein food. Both approaches result in successful weight loss, and selection of a weight management food often is based on personal preference and individual patient factors.[26,58,72,92–97] Effects of time-limited feeding and dietary carbohydrate content on weight loss were studied in overweight, group-housed cats that were free-choice fed a reduced energy, high-fiber, relatively high-carbohydrate food (Hill's Science Diet® Feline Light® Adult Dry).[58] Cats gradually made the transition to food access that was restricted to four hours/day and were randomly assigned to continue the reduced energy food or receive a therapeutic low-carbohydrate food (Purina DM® Feline Formula Dry). On average, when cats had their energy intake restricted to the same degree, they lost weight at the same rate regardless of which food (or amount of dietary protein or carbohydrate) they received.

Recently, there has been increased focus on the role of dietary protein for managing overweight or obese cats. Feeding increased protein (11.1 to 13.6 g/100 kcal) has been associated with greater loss of body fat and less loss of lean body mass compared with lower protein foods (6.9 to 10.5 g/100 kcal).[72,94,98] In contrast, cats eating a low-protein food (7.7 g/100 kcal) lost body weight with no significant change in lean body mass[96] in one study, while cats in another study lost lean body mass (median decrease of 13%) when eating a high-protein food (12 g/100 kcal).[93] One study showed that cats eating less protein (9 g/100 kcal) needed fewer calories to lose and maintain body weight compared with cats eating more protein (11.9 g/100 kcal).[98] In another study, heat production was greater in lean cats during consumption of a high-protein food (11.1 g/100 kcal) compared with lower protein (6.9 g/100 kcal); this difference was not observed in obese cats, however.[72] The authors suggested that increased heat production could result in cats developing less obesity over time when eating a higher protein food. However, this was not supported by another study in which there was no difference in energy expenditure or loss of body fat content when cats were fed a high-protein food (13.3 g/100 kcal) compared with a low-protein food (7.7 g/100 kcal).[96] In addition, cats offered dry food free choice after neutering had significantly greater food intake and body weight gain when fed high-protein (11 g/100 kcal) vs. less protein (7.8 g/100 kcal).[60]

It has been recommended that overweight or obese cats be fed more than 45% protein as calories to maximize fat loss and maintain lean body mass.[99] This recommendation was based in part on results of a study in which beneficial effects occurred in cats fed 45.2 grams of protein/100 grams of food (or 11.1 grams of protein/100 kcal).[72] This amount of protein is found in most therapeutic feline weight management foods manufactured by the major pet food companies (Table 4.6). Based on all available evidence, a variety of dietary protein amounts

Table 4.6. Nutrient content of feline therapeutic weight management/diabetic foods.

Brand/product	Form	Protein (g/100kcal)	Carbs (g/100kcal)	Carbs % ME	Fat (g/100kcal)	Crude fiber (g/100kcal)
Hill's® Prescription Diet® m/d® Feline	Can	13.1	3.9	13	4.8	1.5
Hill's® Prescription Diet® m/d® Feline	Dry	12.2	3.5	12	5.2	1.4
Hill's® Prescription Diet® r/d® with Liver and Chicken Feline	Can	12.3	10.2	35	3	5.0
Hill's® Prescription Diet® r/d® with Chicken Feline	Dry	11.2	9.6	35	2.9	4.1
Hill's® Prescription Diet® w/d® with Chicken Feline	Can	11.5	7.6	25	4.8	3.1
Hill's® Prescription Diet® w/d® with Chicken Feline	Dry	11.5	10.2	36	2.9	2.2
Purina Veterinary Diets® DM Dietetic Management® Feline	Can	9.8	1.4	NR	7.1	0.7
Purina Veterinary Diets® DM Dietetic Management® Feline	Dry	12.9	3.4	13	4	0.3
Purina Veterinary Diets® OM Overweight Management® Feline	Can	13	4.1	NR	4.7	3.9
Purina Veterinary Diets® OM Overweight Management® Feline	Dry	16.6	6.5	23	2.5	1.8
Royal Canin Veterinary Diet® Calorie Control CC™ High Protein	Can	13.6	2.8	11	4.3	0.6
Royal Canin Veterinary Diet® Calorie Control CC™ High Protein	Dry	11.6	8.4	32	2.7	1.1
Royal Canin Veterinary Diet® Calorie Control CC™ High Fiber	Can	9	8.2	29	4.7	2
Royal Canin Veterinary Diet® Calorie Control CC™ High Fiber	Dry	10.4	10.6	37	3.1	4.3
Iams® Veterinary Formula Weight Loss Restricted-Calorie™ Feline	Can	10.2	7.5	21	2.5	0.4
Iams® Veterinary Formula Weight Loss Restricted-Calorie™ Feline	Dry	9.5	12	42	3	0.7
Iams® Veterinary Formula Weight Control Optimum Weight Control	Dry	10.2	10.9	37	3.2	0.4

Carb = carbohydrates; ME = metabolizable energy (calories); NR = not reported have been associated with effective weight loss and maintenance of lean body mass in cats.

> **Key Point**
>
> Foods with a wide range of protein amounts have been associated with effective weight loss.

Veterinary Therapeutic Food vs. Low-carb/High-protein Over-the-counter Food For Diabetic or Overweight Cats

Nutritional recommendations for diabetic or overweight cats should be based on patient and owner factors as well as characteristics of the foods. It is generally assumed that over-the-counter foods are less expensive; however, many of these foods cost more than therapeutic foods sold only by veterinary hospitals. In general, over-the-counter foods are more convenient because they are sold in more outlets where pet owners shop. The disadvantages of some of these foods are that they contain excessive nutrients (e.g., calcium, phosphorus, sodium) and there may be significant variability in nutrient content between products, even between different flavors within the same brand (Table 4.7). This may result in lack of day-to-day consistency in nutrient intake, which is likely an important consideration for diabetic cats. Finally, clinical studies are more often conducted using therapeutic foods; therefore, effectiveness of these products is more likely to be supported by published evidence.

> **Key Point**
>
> Over-the-counter canned foods often contain excessive nutrients, and nutrient content varies significantly, even between different flavors of the same brand.

Summary

Cats are carnivores that have adapted to foods higher in protein; however, they are able to efficiently use appropriately processed carbohydrates found in commercial cat foods.[38,48–50,100] The role of dietary carbohydrates (and dry food) in the pathogenesis of feline diseases, particularly obesity and diabetes mellitus, is a topic of considerable debate. Currently available evidence does not support a direct

Table 4.7. Nutrient information for selected over-the-counter moist feline foods.

Brand/product	Pro % DM	Carb % DM	Carb % ME	Carb g/100 kcal	Ca % DM	Phos % DM	Na % DM
Hill's® Science Diet® Kitten Healthy Development Liver & Chicken Entrée Minced	49	16	13	3.4	1.3	0.95	0.32
Hill's® Science Diet® Kitten Healthy Development Savory Salmon Entrée Minced	49	15	12	3.5	1	0.93	0.36
Hill's® Science Diet® Kitten Healthy Development Turkey and Giblets Entrée Minced	49	16	12	3.3	1	0.93	0.39
Natura EVO® Turkey and Chicken Formula Cat and Kitten Food	47	6.2	–	–	1.8	1.3	0.55
Natura EVO® 95% Duck	40	6	–	–	2.2	1.4	0.35
Nature's Variety Instinct® Venison Grain-Free	36	24	–	–	3.8	2.6	0.55
Purina® Fancy Feast® Flaked Fish and Shrimp Feast	80	0	–	0	1.9	1.6	0.53
Purina® Fancy Feast® Turkey and Giblets Feast®	52	1.7	–	0.35	1.8	1.7	0.68
Purina® Fancy Feast® Chicken Feast in Gravy	61	13	–	3.4	1.3	1.1	1.50
Purina® Fancy Feast® Savory Salmon Feast	56	0	–	0	2.2	2	1
Purina® Pro Plan® Sardines and Tuna Entreé in Aspic	71	0	–	0	3.1	2.2	0.37
Purina® Pro Plan® Selects® Natural Beef and Brown Rice Entreé	50	6	–	1.3	2.9	2.2	0.56

Pro = protein, Carb = carbohydrate, Ca = calcium; Phos = phosphorus; Na = sodium.

cause-and-effect relationship between increased carbohydrate or dry food intake and diabetes mellitus or obesity in cats.[34,37] It is likely that a combination of factors plays a role and that increased dietary carbohydrates is an indirect factor due to free-choice feeding of dry food (which is typically high in carbohydrates) and subsequent obesity, which is associated with insulin resistance. Health care team members must make appropriate recommendations to help pet owners maintain ideal body condition in their cats throughout their lifetimes to decrease occurrence of subsequent diseases.

> **Key Point**
>
> Currently available evidence does not support a direct cause-and-effect relationship between increased carbohydrate or dry food intake and diabetes mellitus or obesity in cats.

Determining How Much to Feed

Combating Portion Distortion

It should come as no surprise that most dogs and cats overeat if they have unlimited access to food. In fact, it has been reported that 30% to 40% of dogs and cats overeat and become overweight or obese when food is available *ad libitum*.[101] It is interesting to note the correlation between those numbers and the estimated prevalence of obesity in pets (40% or more).

Although it is essential to address all aspects of the environment that contribute to obesity (e.g., lack of exercise and behavioral patterns for pets and owners), controlling calorie intake is imperative for a successful weight loss program. Controlling calorie intake is a simple concept to grasp but a difficult one to implement. From the owner's perspective there are perhaps two fundamental barriers to effective control of calorie intake: label confusion and portion distortion.

All therapeutic weight loss food that is labeled as complete and balanced must list feeding directions on the product label. These directions must be expressed in common terms and must appear prominently on the label. Feeding directions should state, "Feed (X/unit of product) per (X weight) of dog (or cat)" and indicate the frequency of feeding. Most therapeutic weight loss foods also indicate the amount to feed for the target body weight.

The only exception to this rule is for products that bear the "use only as directed by your veterinarian" statement. Because the veterinarian will presumably provide proper instruction about feeding of the product, explicit feeding directions are not required. Many veterinary therapeutic/wellness products, however, may still provide specific directions either on the label or in accompanying product literature. Despite the best efforts of manufacturers, these feeding statements are general guidelines at best. Because of individual variation, many animals require more or less food than that recommended on the label to achieve optimal body condition.

While individual variation is an important reason why following feeding directions on packages may not result in weight loss, a more important point is that they are rendered useless because few owners actually read or follow these directions. In a 2002 study of pet owner feeding behaviors, only 6% of pet owners responded that they followed the package label feeding directions when determining how much to feed their pet.[102] Though this number may seem low, it is corroborated by studies on the use of nutritional information on food labels for people. While studies of adult consumers show the reported consumer use of nutritional labels is high, the actual use is considerably lower and most accurately described as infrequent.[103]

If pet owners ignore the instructions on the product labels, how do they decide how much to feed their pet? In one study, the most common way was to "use their own best judgment (Figure 4.8)."[102] Sadly, only 4% reported getting and using a recommendation on the amount to feed their pet from the veterinary health care team.

Unfortunately, most owners' best judgment is not an ideal technique for determining the appropriate amount of food for the pet. This method is fraught with problems, not the least of which is the prevalence of portion size distortion in most U.S. households. In the United States, portion sizes have been increasing since the 1970s; this trend has been

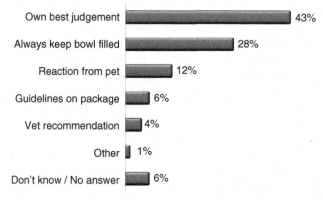

Figure 4.8. Responses of pet owners to the question, "How do you determine how much to feed your pet?" Source: Habits and Practices of Pet Owners: Hill's Pet Nutrition, Inc., 2002.

Table 4.8. Increase in serving size and calories of a typical fast food meal.

| | 1980s | | Today | |
	Serving	Calories	Serving	Calories
Cheeseburger	3 oz	333	8 oz	590
Fries	2.4 oz	210	6.9 oz	610
Soda	6.5 oz	85	20 oz	250
Total Calories		**628**		**1450**

Data from the Department of Health and Human Services website: http://www.nhlbi.nih.gov/health/public/heart/obesity/lose_wt/index.htm

observed in a variety of settings including restaurants, supermarkets, and the home.[104–106] Since the 1970s, marketplace food portions steadily increased in size and currently exceed the recommended standard ones, creating a distorted view of just what constitutes a normal serving size. This increased portion size corresponds with increased consumption of calories. Take, for example, the differences in calorie content of these two similar meals, separated by about 20 years (Table 4.8).

For a 30-year-old woman (height: 5'6", weight: 140 lbs), the 1980s meal represents 31% of her daily caloric needs (approximately 2,000 calories/day). That same meal today provides 72% of her daily requirements. Indeed, portion sizes offered by fast food chains today are two to five times larger than when first introduced.[107] When McDonald's first started in 1955, its only hamburger weighed about 1.6 oz; now, the largest hamburger patty weighs 8 oz, an increase of 500%.[107] This is true for many items, including our morning coffee. When our parents ordered a coffee two decades ago, they were given an 8-oz cup of coffee. Today, most of us feel like we aren't getting our money's worth unless the cup is at least 12 oz, and it's not unusual to see 32-oz coffee cups, four times the size they used to be. When coffee morphs into a mocha, this morning coffee has as many calories as a full meal. Given these changes in what most owners consider a normal portion size for their own meals, it is little wonder that they extrapolate this perception to their pets.

Determine Daily Calorie Requirements

Pet owners need the help of the veterinary health care team if they are going to successfully manage their pet's weight. As discussed in Chapter 2, determining the ideal body weight is the first step in a successful weight management plan. The next step is to calculate the calories required to reach that ideal body weight. Several methods exist for determining the caloric need and thus the quantity of food necessary for weight loss. Four common methods include: product information, calculations based on estimated ideal weight, calculations based on current food intake, and calculations based on current (obese) weight. All of these methods generate estimates. Regardless of which one is used, it should be considered a starting point and adjustments should be made as necessary.

Product Information

The simplest method for determining the amount to feed for weight loss is to obtain the food dose recommendation from the pet food manufacturer. This information may be available on the product label, from published company literature, on the company website, or by using calculators or proprietary software programs. However, the last method often requires an estimate of the patient's ideal or optimal weight. Determination of ideal body weight is discussed in Chapter 2.

Calculations Based on Ideal Body Weight

When a dog or cat is at ideal body weight, about 70% of their daily energy requirement (DER) is used for maintenance of lean body tissue, which is defined as the resting energy requirement (RER). Maintaining adipose tissue in obese pets requires relatively little energy; therefore, most calories consumed by an overweight patient, regardless of the degree of obesity, are used to support lean body tissues. This concept is discussed in detail in Chapter 2 but bears repeating here: Feed the healthy pet inside, not the fat. For dogs and cats, the calories required for RER at optimal weight can be used as an initial estimate of calories required for appropriate weight loss. RER can be obtained directly from Table 2.4 or calculated using one of two equations:

RER (kcal/day) = $70 \times$ (BWkg)$^{0.75}$. This calculation can be performed with a calculator that has a fractional exponent key or by cubing the body weight and taking its square root twice.

RER (kcal/day) = $30 \times$ (BWkg) + 70. Results using this formula correlate well with results derived from the first formula for body weights greater than 2 kg.

This level of restriction should provide a reasonable rate of weight loss; about 1% to 2% loss of obese body weight/week. Because this level of restriction makes caloric intake nearly equal to the calories required to support lean body mass at optimal weight, energy for physical activity must be supplied by catabolizing (burning) fat stores.

Calculations Based on Current Food Intake

This method requires knowledge of the number of calories the pet is currently eating based on information obtained from the diet history, then reducing the calories consumed. This, of course, assumes that a thorough diet history is available. Accurately estimating calorie intake may be difficult if multiple members of the family feed the pet or if treats and people food are offered. This method also requires determining the calorie content of the foods being consumed. Depending on the diet, this may be a cumbersome task.

One option is to use a web-based program to perform calculations based on the current food information obtained from the diet history. One such service is Balance IT (info@dvmconsulting.com), a fee-based program designed to help veterinary health care teams with calculation-based weight-loss feeding plans. The user can select/enter all the foods a patient is currently fed (based on the diet history) and the program then determines the caloric needs of the patient for weight loss. Users can set the desired weight loss rates and select the commercial weight loss food they wish to feed (along with any treats up to 10% of daily calories). The program calculates the amount to feed and enters this information into a report to be printed for clients. Based on weight rechecks, the software adjusts the amount to feed the patient.

This can be an excellent way to calculate the initial food dose if the information in the feeding history is complete and accurate. If the food history is incomplete, the owner can be instructed to return home and record actual amounts fed for a three-day period and either phone in the information or schedule a follow-up visit. Potential limitations of this approach include losing the attention and commitment of the owners due to busy schedules, inaccurate owner reports due to concerns of having been "feeding too much" and having to convert volume measures to calories for a variety of foods.

Calculations Based on Obese Weight

Finally, the current (obese) weight can be used to determine the amount to feed for controlled weight loss. Using the current weight is more straightforward than determining ideal weight. This method also requires a calculation for the amount of desired weekly weight loss. The following steps represent the process for estimating the initial amount to feed for weight loss using obese body weight and a desired rate of weight loss:

1. Obtain current (obese) body weight.
2. Calculate DER for current body weight = estimated current daily energy intake.
3. Calculate the energy content of body fat (7,920 kcal/kg adipose tissue) to be lost weekly, assuming a target weight loss of between 0.5% and 2% initial body weight/week.
4. Divide the weekly amount of adipose calories by seven to obtain desired daily calorie deficit.
5. Subtract the daily calorie deficit from the DER to obtain the number of calories to feed/day.
6. Divide the number of calories to feed/day by the energy density of the selected food to determine the amount of food to feed/day.

Regardless of the method used to calculate calories, this value should be considered a starting point. Individual animals of the same weight have a wide variation of energy requirements. Therefore, in practice, animals will be seen that need the same, markedly fewer and, occasionally, markedly more calories than product literature or calculations suggest. Indeed, caloric restriction based on these initial estimates may be insufficient to produce weight loss or may even produce weight gain in some patients.[108]

Food Dose

After the caloric intake for weight loss is calculated the amount of food to be fed is determined by dividing total calories/day by the calorie content of the selected food. Calorie content of many therapeutic foods is available on the package label. Other sources include manufacturers' product literature and websites. The following is an example using the current obese weight to calculate caloric intake and amount of food to be fed.

An obese dog has a body weight of 30 kg and a BCS of 5/5. The DER for the dog's obese weight is calculated using the formula DER = RER × 1.4. RER (kcal/day) = 30(BWkg) + 70. RER = 30 (30 kg) + 70 = 970 kcal/day. DER = 1.4 × RER = 1.4 × 970 = 1,358 kcal/day.

RER can also be obtained directly from Table 2.4. A targeted weight loss of 1.5% of the dog's obese weight/week is 0.45 kg/week. The energy density of adipose tissue is 7,920 kcal/kg; 7,920 kcal/kg × 0.45 kg = 3,564 kcal/week or 509 kcal/day (3,564 kcal/week ÷ 7 days/ week). The calculated daily energy intake for this rate of weight loss = 1,358 kcal/day – 509 kcal = 849 kcal/day. The food selected for weight loss provides 220 kcal/cup; 849 kcal/day ÷ 220 kcal/cup = 3 and 7/8 cups/day. This amount is a starting point and may need to be modified to achieve the desired weight loss. Recheck body weight after two to three weeks.

This is perhaps the most important step in the nutritional management of obese pets. To increase the effectiveness of weight management programs the veterinary health care team must make a specific recommendation that includes the brand and type of food, the amount of food to be fed each day, and the feeding method to be used.

Summary

When it comes to weight loss products for both humans and pets, sorting out fact from fiction can be challenging. Application of the concepts of evidence-based medicine can assist veterinarians and health care team members in this endeavor. As a group, therapeutic weight loss foods have the best evidence to support their efficacy. Individual supplements have not been shown to increase weight loss consistently or significantly. Providing owners with a specific nutritional recommendation using calculations based on ideal weight will increase the likelihood of success in any weight management program.

In Practice

There are many ways to determine the food dose for a given patient. Many weight management programs fail because the recommended food dose exceeds the caloric requirements for weight loss. Using ideal body weight to determine the food dose minimizes these types of errors. The discrepancy in food dosage that can result from whether a patient with a BCS of 5/5 has 40% body fat or 60% body fat is significant. For example, the following equation can be used to estimate ideal body weight:

$$\text{Ideal weight} = \text{current weight} \times (100 - \text{percent body fat}) \div 0.80$$

If an overweight (5/5) 30-kg dog is assumed to have 40% body fat, its estimated ideal weight is 22.5 kg and its estimated resting energy requirement (RER) would be 745 kcal/day (Table 2.4). However, if that 30-kg (5/5) dog actually has 60% body fat, then the ideal weight is 15 kg and its RER would be 520 kcal/day, a difference of 225 kcal/day. Considering that the average calorie density of most dry canine therapeutic weight loss foods is approximately 235 kcal/cup, underestimating percentage body fat will result in overfeeding by approximately one cup of food/day. For the dog with 60% body fat, a weight loss program based on feeding 745 kcal/day will likely be unsuccessful and lead to frustration for the client and the veterinary health care team.

References

1. Temple NJ. 2010. The marketing of dietary supplements in North America: The emperor is (almost) naked. *J Altern Complement Med* 16:803–806.
2. Roudebush P, Allen TA, Dodd CE, et al. 2004. Application of evidence-based medicine to veterinary clinical nutrition. *J Am Vet Med Assoc* 224:1765–1771.
3. Roudebush P, Schoenherr WD, Delaney SJ. 2008. An evidence-based review of the use of nutraceuticals and dietary supplementation for the management of obese and overweight pets. *J Am Vet Med Assoc* 232:1646–1655.
4. Klomp AE, van de Sluis B, Klomp LW, et al. 2003. The ubiquitously expressed MURR1 protein is absent in canine copper toxicosis. *J Hepatol* 39:703–709.

5. Chan DL. 2008. The role of nutrients in modulating disease. *J Small Anim Pract* 49:266–271.

6. Yamka RM, Friesen KG, Gao X, et al. 2008. The effects of weight loss on gene expression in dogs (Abstract). *Journal of Veterinary Internal Medicine* 22:741.

7. Roudebush P, Schoenherr WD, Delaney SJ. 2008. An evidence-based review of the use of therapeutic foods, owner education, exercise, and drugs for the management of obese and overweight pets. *Journal of the American Veterinary Medical Association* 233:717–725.

8. Burkholder WJ, Bauer JE. 1998. Foods and techniques for managing obesity in companion animals. *J Am Vet Med Assoc* 212:658–662.

9. Burley VJ, Leeds AR, Blundell JE. 1987. The effect of high and low-fibre breakfasts on hunger, satiety and food intake in a subsequent meal. *Int J Obes* 11 Suppl 1:87–93.

10. Stevens J, Levitsky DA, VanSoest PJ, et al. 1987. Effect of psyllium gum and wheat bran on spontaneous energy intake. *Am J Clin Nutr* 46:812–817.

11. Butterwick RF, Markwell PJ, Thorne CJ. 1994. Effect of level and source of dietary fiber on food intake in the dog. *J Nutr* 124:2695S–2700S.

12. Jewell DE, Toll PW. 1996. Effect of fiber on food intake in dogs. *Veterinary Clinical Nutrition* 3:115–188.

13. Greenberg I, Stampfer MJ, Schwarzfuchs D, et al. 2009. Adherence and success in long-term weight loss diets: The dietary intervention randomized controlled trial (DIRECT). *J Am Coll Nutr* 28:159–168.

14. Nackers LM, Ross KM, Perri MG. 2010. The association between rate of initial weight loss and long-term success in obesity treatment: Does slow and steady win the race? *Int J Behav Med* 17:161–167.

15. Blanchard G, Nguyen P, Gayet C, et al. 2004. Rapid weight loss with a high-protein low-energy diet allows the recovery of ideal body composition and insulin sensitivity in obese dogs. *J Nutr* 134:2148S–2150S.

16. Diez M, Nguyen P, Jeusette I, et al. 2002. Weight loss in obese dogs: Evaluation of a high-protein, low-carbohydrate diet. *J Nutr* 132:1685S–1687S.

17. Fritsch DA, Ahle NW, Jewell DE, et al. 2010. A high-fiber food improves weight loss compared to a high-protein, high-fat food in pet dogs in a home setting. *International Journal of Applied Research in Veterinary Medicine* 8:138–145.

18. German AJ, Holden SL, Bissot T, et al. 2007. Dietary energy restriction and successful weight loss in obese client-owned dogs. *J Vet Intern Med* 21:1174–1180.

19. German AJ, Holden SL, Bissot T, et al. 2009. A high protein high fibre diet improves weight loss in obese dogs. *Vet J* 183:294–297.

20. Borne AT, Wolfsheimer KJ, Truett AA, et al. 1996. Differential metabolic effects of energy restriction in dogs using diets varying in fat and fiber content. *Obes Res* 4:337–345.

21. Yamka RM, Frantz NZ, Friesen KG. 2007. Effects of 3 canine weight loss foods on body composition and obesity markers. *International Journal of Applied Research in Veterinary Medicine* 5:125–132.

22. Flint A, Moller BK, Raben A, et al. 2004. The use of glycaemic index tables to predict glycaemic index of composite breakfast meals. *Br J Nutr* 91:979–989.

23. Sunvold GD, Bouchard GF. 1998. The glycemic response of dietary starch. Iams Nutrition Symposium: Recent Advances in Canine and Feline Nutrition 123–131.

24. Flickinger EA, Sunvold GD. 2005. Early nutritional management to reduce the risks of diabetes and obesity. Canine Pediatric Symposium: World Small Animal Veterinary Association.

25. Nguyen P, Dumon H, Biourge V, et al. 1998. Glycemic and insulinemic responses after ingestion of commercial foods in healthy dogs: Influence of food composition. *J Nutr* 128:2654S–2658S.

26. Roudebush P, Schoenherr WD, Delaney SJ. 2008. An evidence-based review of the use of therapeutic foods, owner education, exercise, and drugs for the management of obese and overweight pets. *J Am Vet Med Assoc* 233:717–725.

27. Appleton DJ, Rand JS, Sunvold GD. 2000. Feline Obesity: Pathogenesis and Implications for the Risk of Diabetes. In: Reinhart GA, Carey DP, eds. *Recent Advances in Canine and Feline Nutrition*. Wilmington, Ohio: Orange Frazer Press, 81–90.

28. Fettman MJ, Stanton CA, Banks LL, et al. 1998. Effects of weight gain and loss on metabolic rate, glucose tolerance, and serum lipids in domestic cats. *Res Vet Sci* 64:11–16.

29. Bravata DM, Sanders L, Huang J, et al. 2003. Efficacy and safety of low-carbohydrate diets: a systematic review. *JAMA* 289:1837–1850.

30. Gross LS, Li L, Ford ES, et al. 2004. Increased consumption of refined carbohydrates and the epidemic of type 2 diabetes in the United States: An ecologic assessment. *Am J Clin Nutr* 79:774–779.

31. Bray GA, Nielsen SJ, Popkin BM. 2004. Consumption of high-fructose corn syrup in beverages may play a role in the epidemic of obesity. *Am J Clin Nutr* 79:537–543.

32. Basciano H, Federico L, Adeli K. 2005. Fructose, insulin resistance, and metabolic dyslipidemia. *Nutr Metab (Lond)* 2:5.

33. Foster GD, Wyatt HR, Hill JO, et al. 2010. Weight and metabolic outcomes after 2 years on a low-carbohydrate versus low-fat diet: A randomized trial. *Ann Intern Med*;153:147–157.

34. Buffington C. 2008. Dry foods and risk of disease in cats. *Canadian Veterinary Journal* 49:561–563.

35. Greco DS. 2008. Metabolic syndrome—What is it and why should we care? *Top Companion Anim Med* 23:115.

36. Hodgkins E. 2007. *Your Cat—Simple New Secrets to a Longer, Stronger Life*. New York: St. Martin's Press.

37. Laflamme DP. 2008. Letter to the editor: Cats and carbohydrates. *Top Companion Anim Med* 23:159–160.

38. Zoran DL. 2002. The carnivore connection to nutrition in cats. *J Am Vet Med Assoc* 221:1559–1567.

39. Zoran DL. 2010. The Unique Nutritional Needs of the Cat. In: Ettinger SJ, Feldman EC, eds. *Textbook of Veterinary Internal Medicine*, 7th ed, 652–659.

40. Feldman EC. 2009. Diabetes remission in cats: Which insulin is best? *Compendium Continuing Education for Veterinarians* 31;7(A):1–7.

41. Rand J. 1999. Current understanding of feline diabetes: Part 1, pathogenesis. *J Feline Med Surg* 1:143–153.

42. Rios L, Ward C. 2008. Feline diabetes mellitus: Diagnosis, treatment, and monitoring. *Compend Contin Educ Vet* 30:626–639.

43. Rios L, Ward C. 2008. Feline diabetes mellitus: Pathophysiology and risk factors. *Compend Contin Educ Vet* 30:E1–E7.

44. Vondruska J. 1987. The effect of rat carcass diet on the urinary pH of the cat. *Companion Animal Practice* 1:5–9.

45. Debraekeleer J. 2000. Appendices. *Small Animal Clinical Nutrition*, 4th ed. 1074–1075.

46. Kienzle E. 1994. Effect of carbohydrates on digestion in the cat. *J Nutr* 124:2568S–2571S.

47. Kienzle E. 1994. Blood sugar levels and renal sugar excretion after the intake of high carbohydrate diets in cats. *J Nutr* 124:2563S–2567S.

48. de-Oliveira LD, Carciofi AC, Oliveira MC, et al. 2008. Effects of six carbohydrate sources on cat diet digestibility and postprandial glucose and insulin response. *J Anim Sci* 86:2237–2246.

49. Morris JG, Trudell J, Pencovic T. 1977. Carbohydrate digestion by the domestic cat (*Felis catus*). *Br J Nutr* 37:365–373.

50. Thiess S, Becskei C, Tomsa K, et al. 2004. Effects of high carbohydrate and high fat diet on plasma metabolite levels and on i.v. glucose tolerance test in intact and neutered male cats. *J Feline Med Surg* 6:207–218.

51. Hill's Pet Nutrition I. Habits and Practices Study, 2002.

52. Scarlett JM, Donoghue S, Saidla J, et al. 1994. Overweight cats: Prevalence and risk factors. *Int J Obes Relat Metab Disord* 18 Suppl 1:S22–28.

53. Backus RC, Cave NJ, Keisler DH. 2007. Gonadectomy and high dietary fat but not high dietary carbohydrate induce gains in body weight and fat of domestic cats. *Br J Nutr* 98:641–650.

54. Fettman MJ, Stanton CA, Banks LL, et al. 1997. Effects of neutering on body weight, metabolic rate and glucose tolerance of domestic cats. *Res Vet Sci* 62:131–136.

55. Harper EJ, Stack DM, Watson TD, et al. 2001. Effects of feeding regimens on body weight, composition and condition score in cats following ovariohysterectomy. *J Small Anim Pract* 42:433–438.

56. Kanchuk ML, Backus RC, Calvert CC, et al. 2002. Neutering induces changes in food intake, body weight, plasma insulin and leptin concentrations in normal and lipoprotein lipase-deficient male cats. *J Nutr* 132:1730S-1732S.

57. Martin LJ, Siliart B, Dumon HJ, et al. 2006. Spontaneous hormonal variations in male cats following gonadectomy. *J Feline Med Surg* 8:309–314.

58. Michel KE, Bader A, Shofer FS, et al. 2005. Impact of time-limited feeding and dietary carbohydrate content on weight loss in group-housed cats. *J Feline Med Surg* 7:349–355.

59. Nguyen PG, Dumon HJ, Siliart BS, et al. 2004. Effects of dietary fat and energy on body weight and composition after gonadectomy in cats. *Am J Vet Res* 65:1708–1713.

60. Vester B, Suttera S, Keela T, et al. 2009. Ovariohysterectomy alters body composition and adipose and skeletal muscle gene expression in cats fed a high-protein or moderate-protein diet. *Animal* 3:1287–1298.

61. Villaverde C, Ramsey JJ, Green AS, et al. 2008. Energy restriction results in a mass-adjusted decrease in energy expenditure in cats that is maintained after weight regain. *J Nutr* 138:856–860.

62. Belsito KR, Vester BM, Keel T, et al. 2009. Impact of ovariohysterectomy and food intake on body composition, physical activity, and adipose gene expression in cats. *J Anim Sci* 87:594–602.

63. Russell K, Sabin R, Holt S, et al. 2000. Influence of feeding regimen on body condition in the cat. *J Small Anim Pract* 41:12–17.

64. Hoenig M, Ferguson DC. 2002. Effects of neutering on hormonal concentrations and energy requirements in male and female cats. *Am J Vet Res* 63:634–639.

65. Flynn MF, Hardie EM, Armstrong PJ. 1996. Effect of ovariohysterectomy on maintenance energy requirement in cats. *J Am Vet Med Assoc* 209:1572–1581.

66. Root M. 1995. Early spay-neuter in the cat: Effect on development of obesity and metabolic rate *Vet Clin Nutr* 2:132–134.

67. Miller JC, Colagiuri S. 1994. The carnivore connection: Dietary carbohydrate in the evolution of NIDDM. *Diabetologia* 37:1280–1286.

68. Rand JS, Fleeman LM, Farrow HA, et al. 2004. Canine and feline diabetes mellitus: Nature or nurture? *J Nutr* 134:2072S–2080S.

69. Appleton D, Rand J, Priest J, et al. 2004. Dietary carbohydrate source affects glucose concentrations, insulin secretion, and food intake in overweight cats. *Nutrition Research* 24:447–467.

70. Farrow HA, Rand JS, Sunvold GD. 2002. The effect of high protein, high fat or high carbohydrate diets on postprandial glucose and insulin concentrations in normal cats. *J Vet Intern Med* 16:360 (abstract).

71. Hoenig M, Alexander S, Pazak H. 2000. Effect of a high- and low-protein diet on glucose metabolism and lipids in the cat. *Proc Purina Nutrition Forum* 98–99.

72. Hoenig M, Thomaseth K, Waldron M, et al. 2007. Insulin sensitivity, fat distribution, and adipocytokine response to different diets in lean and obese cats before and after weight loss. *Am J Physiol Regul Integr Comp Physiol* 292:R227–234.

73. Leray V, Siliart B, Dumon H, et al. 2006. Protein intake does not affect insulin sensitivity in normal weight cats. *J Nutr* 136:2028S–2030S.

74. Martin GJ, Rand JS. 1999. Food intake and blood glucose in normal and diabetic cats fed *ad libitum*. *J Feline Med Surg* 1:241–251.

75. Mori A, Sako T, Lee P, et al. 2009. Comparison of three commercially available prescription diet regimens on short-term post-prandial serum glucose and insulin concentrations in healthy cats. *Vet Res Commun* 33:669–680.

76. Verbrugghe A, Hesta M, Van Weyengerg S, et al. 2007. The effect of isoenergetic substitution of energy sources on glucose tolerance and insulin sensitivity in healthy non-obese cats. *J Vet Intern Med* 21:1427–1428 (abstract).

77. Crane SW, Cowell CS, Stout NP, et al. 2010. Commercial Pet Foods. In: Hand M, Thatcher CD, Remillard RL, et al., eds. *Small Animal Clinical Nutrition*, 5th ed. Topeka, KS: Mark Morris Institute, 157–190.

78. Curry DL, Morris JG, Rogers QR, et al. 1982. Dynamics of insulin and glucagon secretion by the isolated perfused cat pancreas. *Comp Biochem Physiol A Comp Physiol* 72:333–338.

79. Kitamura T, Yasuda J, Hashimoto A. 1999. Acute insulin response to intravenous arginine in nonobese healthy cats. *J Vet Intern Med* 13:549–556.

80. Morris JG, Rogers QR. 1989. Comparative Aspects of Nutrition and Metabolism of Dogs and Cats. In: Burger I, Rivers J, eds. *Nutrition of the Dog and Cat: Waltham Symposium Number 7*. Cambridge: Cambridge University Press, 35–66.

81. Slingerland LI, Fazilova VV, Plantinga EA, et al. 2009. Indoor confinement and physical inactivity rather than the proportion of dry food are risk factors in the development of feline type 2 diabetes mellitus. *Vet J* 179:247–253.

82. Marshall R, Rand J. 2004. Insulin glargine and a high protein-low carbohydrate diet are associated with high remission rates in newly diagnosed diabetic cats (abstract). *J Vet Intern Med* 18:401.

83. Marshall RD, Rand JS, Morton JM. 2009. Treatment of newly diagnosed diabetic cats with glargine insulin improves glycaemic control and results in higher probability of remission than protamine zinc and lente insulins. *J Feline Med Surg* 11:683–691.

84. Roomp K, Rand J. 2009. Intensive blood glucose control is safe and effective in diabetic cats using home monitoring and treatment with glargine. *J Feline Med Surg* 11:668–682.

85. Bennett N, Greco D, Peterson M, et al. 2006. Comparison of a low carbohydrate-low fiber diet and a moderate carbohydrate-high fiber diet in the management of feline diabetes mellitus. *J Feline Med Surg* 8:73–84.

86. Frank G, Anderson W, Pazak H, et al. 2001. Use of a high-protein diet in the management of feline diabetes mellitus. *Vet Therap* 2:238–246.

87. Mazzaferro EM, Greco DS, Turner AS, et al. 2003. Treatment of feline diabetes mellitus using an alpha-glucosidase inhibitor and a low-carbohydrate diet. *J Feline Med Surg* 5:183–189.

88. Weaver KE, Rozanski EA, Mahony OM, et al. 2006. Use of glargine and lente insulins in cats with diabetes mellitus. *J Vet Intern Med* 20:234–238.

89. Kirk CA. 2006. Feline diabetes mellitus: Low carbohydrates versus high fiber? *Vet Clin North Am Small Anim Pract* 36:1297–1306, vii.

90. Nelson RW, Scott-Moncrieff JC, Feldman EC, et al. 2000. Effect of dietary insoluble fiber on control of glycemia in cats with naturally acquired diabetes mellitus. *J Am Vet Med Assoc* 216:1082–1088.

91. Hall TD, Mahony O, Rozanski EA, et al. 2009. Effects of diet on glucose control in cats with diabetes mellitus treated with twice daily insulin glargine. *J Feline Med Surg* 11:125–130.

92. Bissot T. 2010. Novel dietary strategies can improve the outcome of weight loss in cats. *J Feline Med Surg* 12(2):104–112.

93. German AJ, Holden S, Bissot T, et al. 2008. Changes in body composition during weight loss in obese client-owned cats: Loss of lean tissue mass correlates with overall percentage of weight lost. *J Feline Med Surg* 10:452–459.

94. Laflamme D, Hannah S. 2005. Increased dietary protein promotes fat loss and reduces loss of lean body mass during weight loss in cats. *Intern J Appl Res Vet Med* 3:62–68.

95. Nguyen P, Dumon H, Martin L, et al. 2002. Weight loss does not influence energy expenditure or leucine metabolism in obese cats. *J Nutr* 132:1649S-1651S.

96. Nguyen P, Leray V, Dumon H, et al. 2004. High protein intake affects lean body mass but not energy expenditure in nonobese neutered cats. *J Nutr* 134:2084S-2086S.

97. Szabo J, Ibrahim WH, Sunvold GD, et al. 2000. Influence of dietary protein and lipid on weight loss in obese ovariohysterectomized cats. *Am J Vet Res* 61:559–565.

98. Vasconcellos RS, Borges NC, Goncalves KN, et al. 2009. Protein intake during weight loss influences the energy required for weight loss and maintenance in cats. *J Nutr* 139:855–860.

99. Zoran DL. 2009. Feline obesity: Recognition and management. *Compend Contin Educ Vet* 31:284–293.

100. Kienzle E. 1993. Carbohydrate metabolism of the cat 2. Digestion of starch. *Journal of Animal Physiology and Animal Nutrition* 69:102–114.

101. National Research Council. 2006. Nutrient requirements of dogs and cats. Washington, DC: Ad Hoc Committee on Dog and Cat Nutrition, 22–26.

102. Habits and Practices of Pet Owners: *Hill's Pet Nutrition*, Inc., 2002.

103. Nørgaard MK, Brunsø K. 2009. Families' use of nutritional information on food labels. *Food Quality and Preference* 20:597–606.

104. Ello-Martin JA, Ledikwe JH, Rolls BJ. 2005. The influence of food portion size and energy density on energy intake: Implications for weight management. *Am J Clin Nutr* 82:236S–241S.

105. Nielsen SJ, Popkin BM. 2003. Patterns and trends in food portion sizes, 1977–1998. *JAMA* 289:450–453.

106. Young LR, Nestle M. 2003. Expanding portion sizes in the US marketplace: implications for nutrition counseling. *J Am Diet Assoc* 103:231–234.

107. Young LR, Nestle M. 2007. Portion sizes and obesity: Responses of fast-food companies. *J Public Health Policy* 28:238–248.

108. Laflamme DP, Kuhlman G, Lawler DF. 1997. Evaluation of weight loss protocols for dogs. *Journal of the American Animal Hospital Association* 33:253–259.

Pharmacotherapy for Management of Canine Obesity

Sharon Campbell, DVM, MS, DACVIM

Traditional weight management programs that involve restricted calorie intake and increased exercise have resulted in variable success rates. A summary of research in this area shows that owner compliance was poor, with a drop-out rate of 25% to 47%.[1-3] One study found that dogs in a controlled environment (laboratory setting) had significantly greater weight loss than client-owned dogs fed the same diet and given the same feeding recommendations.[1] This was also observed by in a subsequent study in which client-owned dogs had a rate of weight loss lower than that of laboratory dogs fed a diet of similar composition.[4] Possible reasons for the difference in weight loss between laboratory-housed dogs and client-owned dogs could be attributed to laboratory dogs' greater energy requirements.[5] Alternatively, owner non-compliance likely has a substantial influence. Approximately 43% of participants in one weight loss study cited lack of time to exercise and feeding foods other than those allowed by the diet protocol as the primary reasons for dropping out.[1] Only 56.67% of the owners were able to adhere to the protocol and complete the study.[1] In a second weight loss study, 89% of the pet owners admitted to not complying with the feeding protocol, either feeding treats or observing that the dogs stole food.[4]

> ### Key Point
>
> Many weight management programs fail because of owner noncompliance.

Practical Weight Management in Dogs and Cats, First Edition. Edited by Todd L. Towell.
© 2011 John Wiley and Sons, Inc. Published 2011 by John Wiley & Sons, Inc.

Even when owners completed the study, as many as 60% of dogs did not reach the goal weight.[2] Success of studies can be improved upon with incentives including free food and/or medical services[1,6] or early education (appropriate food, exercise, and risks of obesity) and active monitoring and follow-up.[4,7] Offering a program that is flexible and accommodates specific owners' abilities to comply with feeding and exercise recommendations also can improve success.[8] Nevertheless, obesity afflicts upwards of 40% of adult dogs despite advances in nutrition and development of programs for obesity management.

As discussed in Chapter 1, dysregulation of adipokines associated with increases in white fat tissue can help explain owner non-compliance. The endocrine changes resulting in abnormal appetite and metabolism could impede owners' attempts to control appetite. Exercise may become difficult because of obesity-related conditions such as heat intolerance and respiratory impairment.[9] Additionally, increased inflammatory mediators associated with obesity either lead to or exacerbate osteoarthritis, which can become an impediment for exercise.[10,11]

Pharmacotherapy is another tool that is available to the veterinarian for obese dogs in which the traditional recommendations of diet and exercise for weight loss are not feasible. A multimodal approach that includes appropriate diet and exercise recommendations along with pharmacotherapy can improve weight loss and weight maintenance in obese dogs. Because appetite and metabolism are dysregulated in obesity, logical targets for pharmacotherapy are appetite suppression, increasing metabolism/thermogenesis, or drugs that affect both.

Key Point

Appetite and metabolism are dysregulated in obesity.

Currently two weight management drugs are approved for dogs. Slentrol® (dirlotapide, Pfizer Animal Health) has been approved in the United States, Canada, and the European Union (EU). Yarvitan® (mitratapide, Janssen Animal Health) is approved in the EU. Slentrol® is indicated for the management of obesity in the dog in the U.S. and Canada. Slentrol® and Yarvitan® are approved as an aid in the management of overweight and obesity in adult dogs in the EU. Both drugs should be used as part of an overall weight management program that includes appropriate dietary and exercise considerations.

The advantage of pharmacotherapy in weight management is that it allows the dog to reach the goal weight while controlling appetite sufficiently to aid owner compliance. This was demonstrated in the dirlotapide study, in which weight loss was observed in dogs on dirlotapide that had previously failed food restriction and exercise programs only.[12] As with any weight loss/management program, owner education on appropriate feeding and exercise to maintain a healthy body weight after the drug is discontinued is critical to the success of pharmacotherapy for control of obesity.

Key Point

Pharmacotherapy controls appetite to aid owner compliance.

Mechanism of Action

Dirlotapide and mitratapide are both microsomal triglyceride transfer protein (MTP) inhibitors. During normal digestion and absorption, ingested fat is broken down to free fatty acids and monoglycerides, which are absorbed across the luminal side of the enterocyte, then packaged into chylomicrons within the endoplasmic reticulum before being absorbed into the lymphatic vessels. MTP is the enzyme responsible for packaging the free fatty acid and monoglycerides molecules into chylomicrons. This process delays the fat molecules from moving out of the enterocyte, resulting in a temporary build-up.[13–16] This build-up of fatty acids is thought to cause the release of gut hormones such as peptide YY (PYY) that trigger the satiety center in the hypothalamus, resulting in reduced appetite.[17]

Dirlotapide and mitratapide are partial, potent MTP inhibitors with effects on the enterocyte, which results in an increased delay in processing monoglycerides and free fatty acid into chylomicrons, a greater than normal retention of these fat molecules in the enterocyte, and in the case of dirlotapide, a prolonged secretion of PYY (Figure 5.1). This class of drugs leads to weight loss by decreased fat absorption from the enterocyte and appetite suppression. Dirlotapide weight loss effects are 90% due to appetite suppression and 10% to decreased fat absorption.[14] Mitratapide effects are attributed primarily to decreased fat absorption with minimal appetite suppression.[16] The reduction in appetite by mitratapide is linked to the local mode of action at the level of the gut, inhibition of uptake of dietary lipids, and distribution in the enterocytes, which triggers a negative feedback signal on feed intake. Increased

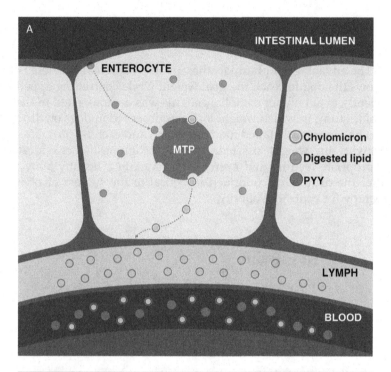

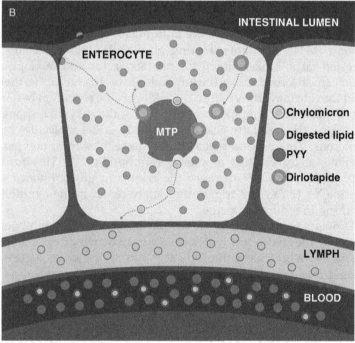

Figure 5.1. Proposed dirlotapide mechanism of action. A. During normal absorption of digested fat, the presence of intestinal lipids triggers the release of hormones, such as peptide YY (PYY), secreted by endocrine cells. When circulating PYY reaches the hypothalamus, it acts as a satiety signal. B. Partial inhibition of MTP prevents some of the lipid from being packaged into chylomicrons for absorption into lymphatics. As a result, digested lipids accumulate in the enterocyte. The higher concentration of lipids in the enterocyte causes higher, constant levels of circulating PYY in the bloodstream. Weight loss is attributed to a combination of decreased fat absorption and decreased appetite and food consumption. Courtesy Pfizer Animal Health.

fat in feces is generally associated with digested fat contained in sloughed enterocytes.

Dirlotapide and mitratapide are rapidly absorbed after oral administration and are highly protein bound. Bioavailability of dirlotapide ranged from 24% to 41% in fed dogs and 22% in fasted dogs.[18] Dirlotapide is metabolized to several metabolites; however, activity of the specific metabolites have not been evaluated.[19] Bioavailability of mitratapide ranged from 55% to 69%, and three active metabolites of mitratapide have been identified.[16] Excretion for both drugs is mainly via the feces. Intravenous administration of dirlotapide had no effect on weight loss, indicating that the local effects of the drug after oral administration are responsible for decreased fat absorption and appetite suppression.[19]

Dosing

Slentrol®

Slentrol® is indicated for obese dogs.[13,20] It should not be administered to cats and is not for use in humans. Slentrol® is supplied as a 5-mg/ml active dirlotapide in an oral solution of medium chain triglycerides. Label recommendation for administration is listed for two distinct treatment phases: weight loss phase and weight management phase. The dose is adjusted to achieve weight loss of 3% body weight/month during the weight loss phase. This rate is rapid enough to encourage pet owners to continue with the treatment[21] while allowing for loss of fat tissue instead of lean tissue, which promotes sustained weight loss.[22] Once the target or goal weight has been attained, the Slentrol® dose is adjusted to provide appetite control and an opportunity for the dog owner to become aware of the appropriate amount of food required to maintain the goal weight.[23] The dosing schedule for Slentrol® administration is listed below and shown in Figure 5.2.

Dosing During Weight Loss Phase
The initial dosage is 0.023 mg/lb (0.05 mg/kg) body weight (BW) once daily for 14 days, then increased to 0.046 mg/lb (0.10 mg/kg) BW once daily for the next 14 days. Dogs should be weighed monthly and the dosage adjusted to maintain a target percent weight loss of greater than or equal to 3%/month from the last visit.

If the dog has gained weight or lost less than 3% body weight/month since the last visit, increase the dose by 100% at the first dose increase and then by 50% each subsequent month as necessary. Dosage increases for dogs that do not achieve the monthly target weight loss of more than 3% body weight should continue until the dog reaches the desired goal weight.

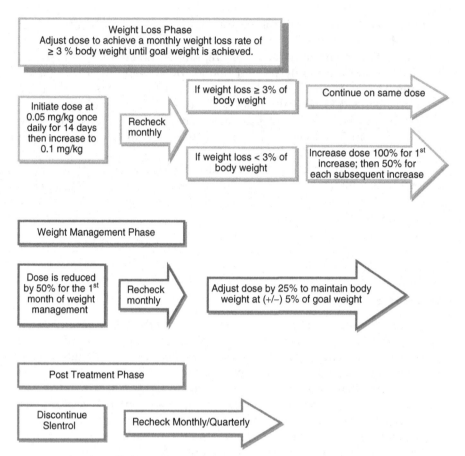

Figure 5.2. Slentrol® dosing schedule.

Dosage During Weight Management Phase

A three-month weight management phase is recommended to success-fully maintain weight loss achieved with treatment. During this phase, Slentrol® dosing is continued at a reduced dose to aid in determining the optimal level of food intake and physical activity required to main-tain the goal weight.

The dose is reduced by 50% for the first month of the weight manage-ment phase, with the intent of maintaining the weight within ± 5% of the goal weight (weight achieved at the end of the weight loss period). At the subsequent monthly rechecks, the dose can be adjusted by 25% to stay within ± 5% of goal weight.

Slentrol® can be administered with or without food. The maximum dose that may be administered is 0.45 mg/lb (1 mg/kg) daily. Manufacturers provide syringes for dosing. The maximum duration of treatment is 12 months. When Slentrol® is discontinued, appetite suppression persists for approximately two days.[14] After discontinua-

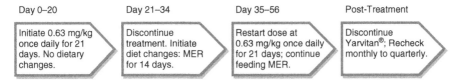

Day 0–20	Day 21–34	Day 35–56	Post-Treatment
Initiate 0.63 mg/kg once daily for 21 days. No dietary changes.	Discontinue treatment. Initiate diet changes: MER for 14 days.	Restart dose at 0.63 mg/kg once daily for 21 days; continue feeding MER.	Discontinue Yarvitan®; Recheck monthly to quarterly.

Figure 5.3. Yarvitan® dosing schedule. Dosage on days 1 and 35 should be calculated based on the dog's current body weight. MER = maintenance energy requirement.

tion of Slentrol®, some dogs may experience polyphagia and regain weight, which emphasizes the need for proper dietary management after discontinuation of the drug.

Yarvitan®

Yarvitan® is supplied as a 5-mg/ml active mitratapide in an oral solution of Macrogol 400, sucralose for flavoring, and butylated hydroxyanisole as an antioxidant.[16] The label provides recommendations for three distinct treatment phases: an initial three-week treatment phase, a two-week non-treatment phase that includes a nutritional program, and a three-week treatment phase that includes continuation of the nutritional program.

Dosing during drug administration (phases 1 and 3) is 0.63 mg/kg; dosing is based on the current body weight of the dog. The drug must be administered with food. Optimal efficacy is obtained when Yarvitan® is administered together with food. No effect on appetite suppression was seen when Yarvitan® was administered with a low-fat diet (5.5% DMB fat content). Yarvitan® administration should be restricted to one treatment course/dog. Yarvitan® is an initial step in an obesity management program. It must be combined with changes in diet, which must be continued after treatment is finished (Figure 5.3).[16] Manufacturers provide pipettes for dosing.

Clinical Response

The Slentrol® and Yarvitan® clinical studies involving client-owned dogs were multi-center, blinded, randomized, and placebo controlled. Both drugs effectively decreased body weight. However, comments regarding comparative efficacy cannot be made due to the difference in study design, dosing, and whether or not dietary restrictions were included as part of the weight loss program.

Slentrol® Efficacy Summary

A total of four multi-center, blinded, placebo-controlled, randomized clinical studies (studies A to D) conducted in the EU and U.S. confirmed

Slentrol® efficacy for weight loss and weight maintenance in obese dogs (U.S.) or overweight and obese dogs (EU).[12,24] Placebo-treated dogs received corn oil administered at volume doses that varied by study (0.01 ml/kg or 0.4 ml/kg) and were equivalent to the volume (ml) dosage of dirlotapide. Volume doses were adjusted according to percentage change in body weight over the course of the study. The initial dosage of dirlotapide varied for the studies. In all studies, dogs were examined at approximately 28-day intervals and dose adjustments were made as required to allow weight loss at approximately 3% of body weight/month up to a maximum dosage of 1 mg/kg. Previous studies have shown that a 1% to 2% rate of weight loss/week results in loss of fat tissue rather than lean tissue.[14]

The dosing duration also varied by study, with dogs receiving dirlotapide or placebo for a weight loss phase of four or six months. In studies that included a weight maintenance phase, dogs that achieved the target body weight received dirlotapide or a placebo at a dosage to maintain body weight for an additional two to three months and were followed for up to two months after dirlotapide was discontinued (post-treatment phase). Dogs were required to receive nutritionally balanced diets and treats according to American Association of Feed Control Officials (AFFCO) standards. No other restrictions on amount or type of food or treats were required. The study design for each of the four studies is shown in Table 5.1.

Dogs in the dirlotapide-treated groups had a mean weight change of –11.8% to –15.9% during the weight loss phase, compared to an average weight loss of –3.0% to –5.3% in the control groups. In all studies, the dirlotapide-treated dogs had greater weight loss than the control groups (P = 0.0001) based on total percent weight change during weight loss phase for U.S. studies or percent weekly weight change for EU studies. The mean percent weight change during the weight loss phase for all studies is shown in Table 5.2, and the percent weight loss for all phases of the studies is shown in Figures 5.4 and 5.5. Mild weight loss continued during the weight maintenance phase (mean weight change –1.5% to –5.3%). During the post-treatment phase, dogs experienced a mild increase in weight, a mean weight change of 2.6% to 3.5%.

Yarvitan® Clinical Efficacy

Two multi-center, blinded, placebo-controlled, randomized clinical studies were conducted in the EU and U.S. that confirmed the efficacy of Yarvitan® in weight loss in obese dogs.[25] The number of dogs enrolled in the U.S. and EU studies was not available. Both studies were conducted according to the label dosing recommendation of a three-week treatment period at 0.63 mg/kg current body weight once daily followed by a two-week treatment-free, calorie-restricted period and then a second three-week treatment period during which mitratipide was

Table 5.1. Study designs for Slentrol®, U.S. and EU Studies[1,2].

Study	Phase	Criteria	Duration	Dosage
Study A (U.S.)	Weight loss	BCS of 8 or 9	16 weeks	Slentrol®: Initial dosage of 0.2 mg/kg once daily, then adjusted monthly to achieve a 3%/month weight loss Control: 0.04 ml/kg once daily, then adjusted monthly to achieve a 3%/month weight loss
	Weight management	Minimum weight loss of 8% by the end of the weight loss period	12 weeks	Slentrol®: Adjusted to keep weight at ±5% of weight at the end of the weight-loss period Controls: N/A. No controls attained the minimum weight loss
	Post treatment		8 weeks	None
Study B (U.S.)	Weight loss	BCS of 8 or 9	16 weeks	Slentrol®: Initial dosage of 0.05 mg/kg once daily for 14 days, then increased to 0.1 mg/kg once daily for the next 14 days; adjusted monthly to achieve a 3%/month weight loss Control: 0.01 ml/kg once daily for 14 days, increased to 0.2 ml/kg once daily for the next 14 days; adjusted monthly to achieve a 3.0%/month weight loss
Study C (EU)	Weight loss	BCS of 6 to 9	Up to 28 weeks	Slentrol®: Initial dosage of 0.05mg/kg once daily for 14 days, then increased to 0.1 mg/kg once daily for the next 14 days; adjusted monthly to achieve a 3%/month weight loss Control: 0.01ml/kg once daily for 14 days, increased to 0.2 ml/kg once daily for the next 14 days; adjusted monthly to achieve a 3%/month weight loss (Continued)

139

Table 5.1. *Continued*

Study	Phase	Criteria	Duration	Dosage
	Weight management	Minimum weight loss of 5% by day 84	12 weeks	Slentrol®: Adjusted to keep weight at ±3% of weight at the end of the weight loss period. Controls: Dose volume increased by 2 × or decreased by 50% to maintain weight at ±5% of weight at end of weight loss period
	Post treatment		4 weeks	None
Study D (EU)	Weight Loss	BCS of 6 to 9	Up to 28 weeks	Slentrol®: Initial dosage of 0.05mg/kg once daily for 14 days, then increased to 0.1 mg/kg once daily for the next 14 days; adjusted monthly to achieve a 3%/month weight loss. Control: 0.01 ml/kg once daily for 14 days, increased to 0.2 ml/kg once daily for the next 14 days; then adjusted monthly to achieve a 3%/month weight loss
	Weight management	Minimum weight loss of 0.35%/week by day 112	12 weeks	Slentrol®: Adjusted to keep weight at ±3% of weight at the end of the weight loss period. Controls: Dose volume increased or decreased by 50% to maintain weight at ±3% of weight at end of weight loss period
	Post treatment		4 weeks	None

BCS = body condition score using an established nine-point scale published as Development and Validation of a Body Condition Score System for Dogs, Laflamme DP, 1997. *Canine Practice* 22:10–15.
1. Gossellin J, McKelvie J, Sherington J, et al. 2007. An evaluation of dirlotapide to reduce body weight of client-owned dogs in two placebo-controlled clinical studies in Europe. *J Vet Pharmacol Ther* 30 Suppl 1:73–80.
2. Wren JA, Ramudo AA, Campbell SL, et al. 2007. Efficacy and safety of dirlotapide in the management of obese dogs evaluated in two placebo-controlled, masked clinical studies in North America. *Journal of Veterinary Pharmacology and Therapeutics* 30:81–89.

Table 5.2. Mean percentage weight change for dogs treated with dirlotapide or a placebo after 112 days of weight loss in U.S. and EU clinical field studies.

Treatment	Mean % weight change Day 0 to 112		Mean % weight change Day 0 up to 196	
Dirlotapide	Study A (U.S.) −14% (95% CI −15.9 to −12.1) N = 41	Study B (U.S.) −11% (95% CI −13 to −10.5) N = 141	Study C (EU) −15% (±8.3) N = 57	Study D (EU) −11% (±8) N = 141
Placebo	−3% (95% CI −5.9 to −0.1) N = 18	−3.9% (95% CI −5.4 to −2.5) N = 74	−5.3% (±7.4) N = 106	−1.7% (±4.7) N = 74

CI: Confidence interval
N: Number of dogs included in analysis

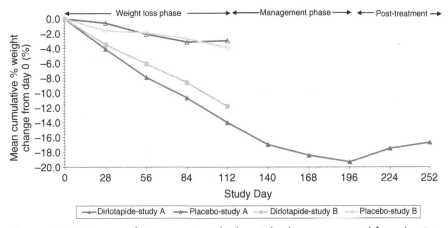

Figure 5.4. Mean cumulative percentage body weight change, measured from day 0 to each scheduled visit for dogs treated with dirlotapide or placebo during U.S. studies.

administered at 0.63 mg/kg current body weight once daily while the dogs remained on a restricted calorie diet.

In both field studies, significant weight loss was achieved in treated animals compared to those that received the placebo, with a mean weight reduction of 6% to 7% over the total treatment period (56 days). In the U.S. study, 22.5% of dogs that received Yarvitan® lost 10% or more body weight compared to 9.5% of the controls. The majority of the weight loss was in the first 21-day treatment period. The body weight remained stable during the treatment-free, calorie-restricted period, with a smaller decrease in body weight during the second treatment

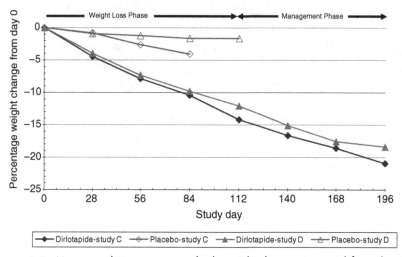

Figure 5.5. Mean cumulative percentage body weight change, measured from day 0 to each scheduled visit for dogs treated with dirlotapide or placebo during EU studies.

period. The extent of weight loss from the treatment-free, calorie-restricted period to the end of the second treatment period was similar in both the control and mitratapide-treated groups. In the U.S. study, the criterion for success was 13% or greater reduction in body weight, and a statistically significantly greater number of dogs that received Yarvitan® reached this criterion, although the number or percent of dogs was not reported.

In the EU study, 25.2% of dogs that received Yarvitan® lost 10% or more body weight compared to 6.8% of the controls. During the two-week calorie restriction period, 53.2% of the placebo-treated dogs and 38.9% of the Yarvitan®-treated dogs gained weight. Increased insulin sensitivity along with weight loss is another effect of Yarvitan®, which has been shown in a laboratory study.[26]

Safety Profile

Prior to using a pharmacotherapeutic agent to treat obesity, dogs should be evaluated for underlying causes of obesity such as hyperadrenocorticism, hypothyroidism, or diabetes mellitus. If present, these chronic diseases should be well controlled prior to initiating any drug therapy.[13,15,16,20,25]

The most commonly reported adverse events in clinical studies for dirlotapide and mitratapide include vomiting, diarrhea/loose stools, lethargy, and anorexia. Signs were mild to moderate, most common during the first month, and typically resolved without treatment. In clinical use of these drugs, if signs persist for more two days, the drug should be discontinued and veterinary intervention sought.

Serum chemistry changes noted for both dirlotapide and mitratapide include increased serum alanine-aminotrasferase (ALT) and aspartate transaminase (AST), and decreased cholesterol, total protein, albumin, globulin, calcium, and alkaline phosphatase (ALP) values. Changes in liver enzymes were not associated with hepatic dysfunction. Elevations in ALT and AST were mild to moderate, remained stable or decreased during the treatment period, and typically returned to normal after cessation of treatment.

If AST or ALT concentrations are markedly elevated, continue to rise during treatment, or are associated with increases in bilirubin and/or ALP, treatment should be discontinued and alternative causes for changes in liver enzymes should be pursued.[13,16,20] Other drug-specific laboratory changes include increased potassium (mitratapide), decreased triglycerides (mitratapide), and decreased high density lipoproteins (dirlotapide).

A number of drugs have been administered concurrently with both drugs and no drug-drug interactions have been reported. Concurrent use with long-term glucocorticoids is contraindicated due to the potential for a combined catabolic effect of weight loss and glucocorticoids.

Effects on Fat-soluble Vitamins

Although plasma levels of vitamin E and A were decreased in a dose-related manner after three months of dirlotapide administration, serum levels were generally above levels previously associated with clinical signs of deficiency. Additionally, vitamin A and E tissue levels were reduced approximately 50% and 20%, respectively, below levels of the control after 12 months of dirlotapide treatment. However, vitamin E levels in adipose tissue were not decreased and both vitamin A and E serum levels returned to normal one month after cessation of treatment.[23] Mitratapide caused decreased absorption of vitamin A and E, but plasma levels were within normal limits. No bleeding abnormalities, which can be indicative of Vitamin K deficiency, were noted. It is unlikely that effects on fat-soluble vitamins will become clinically relevant for either drug when used according to label recommendations.[16,20]

Contraindications, Warnings, Precautions

The contraindications, warnings, precautions for both Slentrol® and Yarvitan® are similar and include:[13,16,20,25]

- Not for use in dogs with impaired liver function or receiving long-term corticosteroid therapy.
- Yarvitan® should not be used in any dog with a history of hypersensitivity to active product or excipients.
- Neither drug has been evaluated in breeding pregnant or lactating dogs or dogs less than 1 year of age (Slentrol®) or 18 months of age (Yarvitan®)
- Pre-existing endocrine disease, hypothyroidism or hyperadrenocorticism, should be managed prior to use.
- **Not for human use under any circumstances. If accidental exposure occurs, seek medical attention.**
- Slentrol® is contraindicated for use in cats because it increases the risk of hepatic lipidosis during weight loss in obese cats.

Implementing a Successful Weight Loss Program Using MTP-Inhibitors

Pharmacotherapy is not required if a dog owner can effectively attain and maintain the established goal weight for her dog with diet and exercise alone. Often, pet owners may want to see if they can be successful with out pharmaceutical intervention. If this is the case, a time limit should be set on how long the owner has to be successful with calorie restriction/exercise program, typically one to two months. This allows for adjustment to the dog's individual metabolic energy requirements (MER) and gives the owner time to realize specific challenges that may arise.

Prior to use of any pharmacotherapeutic agent for control or treatment of obesity, underlying causes or conditions associated with obesity such as hyperadrenocorticism, hypothyroidism, or diabetes mellitus should be diagnosed and well controlled. Once the decision is made to start pharmacotherapy, it is important to recognize that the drug is just one tool that can lead to successful weight loss. The predisposing factors that contributed to the dog's obese state must be addressed. The owner must be re-educated on feeding and exercise to appropriately maintain weight loss after drug cessation. Table 5.3 lists 10 tips for successful weight loss with an MTP-Inhibitor. Some specific considerations:

- Rule out underlying conditions such as hypothyroidism, hyperadrenocorticism, or diabetes mellitus prior to initiating Slentrol® or Yarvitan®.
- A diet change is not required for dogs receiving a nutritionally balanced diet for Slentrol® use. However, better appetite control may be achieved in diets that are not restricted in fat.
- If a diet change is indicated, the new diet should be started at least two weeks prior to initiating the drug to allow for adjustment to the

Table 5.3. Topics for discussion at each monthly weigh-in.

Diseases associated with obesity and benefits of weight loss	
How to assess obesity using body condition scoring and girth measurements	
Keeping a journal	
Discussion about best food for the patient and how to read a dog food label	
Changing the "food is love" paradigm; providing alternative ways to interact with the dog	Playing games (indoor and outdoor activities) Brushing and grooming Old dogs can learn new tricks
Getting the family involved	
Increasing activity; exercise is fun!	Provide a list of local dog-friendly parks Review rules and provide safety tips for walking in a park Discuss pros and cons of doggie day care Find an exercise buddy Create a fitness calendar
Suggest rehabilitation if the dog has a specific condition that limits walking or exercising	
Discussion on giving treats	How much What kind Low-calorie alternatives Various devices that prolong the treat experience Non-food treats Homemade healthy treats
Calories and metabolism	Calculate Relate to diet Relate to exercise
Expectations to keep weight off	Review dog's progress Discuss effect of weight loss on the dog
Taking responsibility: Is the owner the problem or solution?	

new diet and to differentiate between signs associated with change of diet and drug intolerance.

- Higher doses of Slentrol® are required for weight loss with diets that are low in fat; effective dose levels are achieved by following the dosing regime on the label.[13,23] Yarvitan® has been shown to have no effect on appetite with low-fat diets (below 5.5% DMB fat).[16]
- An appropriate rate of weight loss should be maintained.
- As soon as possible, make regular exercise part of the dog's routine because increased exercise leads to increased muscle mass and subsequently increased metabolic rate.
  a. Caution over-enthusiastic owners; initially the exercise should start at a level and duration that the patient and owner can routinely commit to and gradually increase over time.
  b. Exercise should be consistent and daily to avoid the weekend warrior syndrome.

    c. Provide names and locations of local rehabilitation facilities if the dog has a specific injury or conditions that limit exercise
- Use materials provided by the manufacturer, including:
  - a. Journal
  - b. E-mail reminders
  - c. Measuring cup
  - d. Advice on nutrition, healthy treats, fun activities

Addressing Potential Problems

A few clients may consider discontinuing the drug prematurely. It is important that they feel comfortable discussing their concerns with a member of the health care team, which is why a weight management champion is necessary. The ability to get clients back on track depends upon successful communication to address concerns and issues and a program that is flexible for owners and pets.

References

1. Carciofi AC, Venturelli Goncalves KN, Vasconcellos RS, et al. 2005. A weight loss protocol and owners' participation in the treatment of canine obesity. *Ciência Rural* 35:1331–1338.
2. Gentry SJ. 1993. Results of the clinical use of a standardized weight-loss program in dogs and cats. *Journal of the American Animal Hospital Association* 28:369–375.
3. Yaissle JE, Holloway C, Buffington CA. 2004. Evaluation of owner education as a component of obesity treatment programs for dogs. *J Am Vet Med Assoc* 224:1932–1935.
4. German AJ, Holden SL, Bissot T, et al. 2007. Dietary energy restriction and successful weight loss in obese client-owned dogs. *J Vet Intern Med* 21:1174–1180.
5. Hill RC. 2006. Challenges in measuring energy expenditure in companion animals: A clinician's perspective. *J Nutr* 136:1967S–1972S.
6. Saker KE, Remillard RL. 2005. Performance of a canine weight-loss program in clinical practice. *Vet Ther* 6:291–302.
7. Gossellin J, Wren JA, Sunderland SJ. 2007. Canine obesity: An overview. *J Vet Pharmacol Ther* 30 Suppl 1:1–10.
8. Laflamme DP. 2005. Nutrition for aging cats and dogs and the importance of body condition. *Vet Clin North Am Small Anim Pract* 35:713–742.
9. Bach JF, Rozanski EA, Bedenice D, et al. 2007. Association of expiratory airway dysfunction with marked obesity in healthy adult dogs. *Am J Vet Res* 68:670–675.
10. Impellizeri JA, Tetrick MA, Muir P. 2000. Effect of weight reduction on clinical signs of lameness in dogs with hip osteoarthritis. *Journal of the American Veterinary Medical Association* 216:1089–1091.

11. Kealy RD, Lawler DF, Ballam JM, et al. 2002. Effects of diet restriction on life span and age-related changes in dogs. *Journal of the American Veterinary Medical Association* 220:1318–1320.

12. Wren JA, Ramudo AA, Campbell SL, et al. 2007. Efficacy and safety of dirlotapide in the management of obese dogs evaluated in two placebo-controlled, masked clinical studies in North America. *Journal of Veterinary Pharmacology and Therapeutics* 30:81–89.

13. Slentrol. Freedom of Information Summary (FOI). In: Food and Drug Administration CfVMF, CVM, ed: NADA 141–260, 12/DEC/06.

14. Wren JA, King VL, Campbell SL, et al. 2007. Biologic activity of dirlotapide, a novel microsomal triglyceride transfer protein inhibitor, for weight loss in obese dogs. *J Vet Pharmacol Ther* 30 Suppl 1:33–42.

15. Wren JA, King VL, Krautmann MJ, et al. 2007. The safety of dirlotapide in dogs. *J Vet Pharmacol Ther* 30 Suppl 1:43–54.

16. Yarvitan. Summary of Product Characteristics (SPC). In: (EPAR) EPAR, ed: European Medicines Agency (EMEA), 31/Oct/08.

17. Batterham RL, Cohen MA, Ellis SM, et al. 2003. Inhibition of food intake in obese subjects by peptide YY3–36. *N Engl J Med* 349:941–948.

18. Merritt DA, Lynch MP, King VL. 2007. Pharmacokinetics of dirlotapide in the dog. *J Vet Pharmacol Ther* 30 Suppl 1:24–32.

19. Merritt DA, Bessire AJ, Vaz AD, et al. 2007. Absorption, distribution, metabolism, and excretion of dirlotapide in the dog. *J Vet Pharmacol Ther* 30 Suppl 1:17–23.

20. Slentrol. Package Insert: Pfizer Animal Health, October, 2006.

21. Burkholder WJ, Bauer JE. 1998. Foods and techniques for managing obesity in companion animals. *J Am Vet Med Assoc* 212:658–662.

22. Laflamme DP, Kuhlman G. 1995. The effect of weight loss regimen on subsequent weight maintenance in dogs. *Nutrition Research* 15:1019–1028.

23. Gosselin J, Peachey S, Sherington J, et al. 2007. Evaluation of dirlotapide for sustained weight loss in overweight Labrador retrievers. *J Vet Pharmacol Ther* 30 Suppl 1:55–65.

24. Gosselin J, McKelvie J, Sherington J, et al. 2007. An evaluation of dirlotapide to reduce body weight of client-owned dogs in two placebo-controlled clinical studies in Europe. *J Vet Pharmacol Ther* 30 Suppl 1:73–80.

25. Yarvitan. Scientific Discussion. In: (EPAR) EPAR, ed: European Medicines Agency (EMEA), 31/OCT/08.

26. Dobenecker B, De Bock M, Engelen M, et al. 2009. Effect of mitratapide on body composition, body measurements and glucose tolerance in obese Beagles. *Vet Res Commun* 33:839–847.

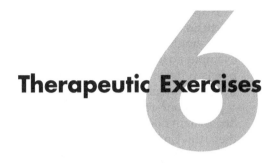

Therapeutic Exercises

Denis J. Marcellin-Little, DEDV, DACVS, DECVS, DACVSMR

Exercises are periods of activity that usually involve repetitive motion such as walking or climbing steps. Exercises are called "therapeutic" when their nature, intensity, frequency, and duration are controlled for specific purposes. Physical activity is a fundamental aspect of the weight management of dogs and cats because it is the only practical strategy that increases energy expenditure. In addition, physical activity may help maintain or increase mobility. This chapter discusses the principles and practical implementation of therapeutic exercises in dogs and cats.

The Principles of Therapeutic Exercises for Dogs and Cats

The Goals of Exercising Dogs

Exercise positively impacts the emotional well-being and the body of dogs. The purposes of exercise include playing, releasing energy, training for a specific working or sporting activity, decreasing the impact of a disease, enhancing recovery after an injury, maintaining fitness, and losing weight. The purposes and benefits of specific exercises and the purposes of exercising in general should be discussed with owners before these exercises are initiated.

Exercises should be adapted to the dog's age, body conformation, fitness level, the local atmospheric conditions (temperature, humidity), and the purpose of the exercises. Skeletally immature dogs are at

Practical Weight Management in Dogs and Cats, First Edition. Edited by Todd L. Towell.
© 2011 John Wiley and Sons, Inc. Published 2011 by John Wiley & Sons, Inc.

increased risk of injury during physical activity, including growth plate fractures and avulsion fractures of ligaments and tendons; therefore, they should be exercised with moderation. Racing greyhounds, for example, go through a breaking-in period after one year of age and start intensive training afterward. They do not race until they are approximately 18 months of age.

Body conformation should be considered as exercise is selected for dogs. Giant dog breeds, for example, are vulnerable to toe injuries when they run. Unfit dogs should be exercised with moderation, particularly in hot climates. Exercise should also be adapted to the needs of a patient. Basic conditioning exercises are ideal for an overweight patient with poor conditioning, but strenuous exercises are suboptimal because they generally carry a higher risk of injury. Furthermore, poorly conditioned dogs can only perform strenuous exercises for brief periods of time and most exercises do not provide physical benefits when performed for brief periods.

The overall goals of an exercise program should guide the decisions regarding the type, duration, intensity, and frequency of exercise for each dog. The owner should be given information that highlights the risks and benefits of each exercise (Table 6.1).

Basic Exercise Parameters

Exercise parameters include the type, frequency, duration, and intensity of exercise. Exercise surfaces and atmospheric parameters (temperature,

Table 6.1. The benefits and risks of selected canine exercises.

Activity	Benefit	Risks
Walking	Strengthens limbs and core	Few (motor vehicle accidents)
	Promotes use of all limbs	
	Weight loss	
Retrieving	Rapidly expends energy	High risk of orthopedic injury
Static exercises (weight shifting)	Promotes use of all limbs, stretching	Minor risk of falls
Obstacle courses (Cavaletti rails)	Promotes use of all limbs, stretching	Minor risk of falls
Walking (underwater treadmill)	Permits exercise with decreased weight bearing	Few (drowning, if unsupervised)
	Promotes limb use	
	Weight loss	
Swimming	Nonweight bearing exercise	Few (drowning, if unsupervised)
	Increases cardiovascular fitness	
	Weight loss	

humidity, daylight) also should be considered. Few studies have compared the relative benefits of exercises in companion animals.[1] The baseline frequency for exercise should be once daily. Longer or more intense exercise sessions should occur at regular intervals (i.e., Wednesday and Sunday rather than Saturday and Sunday).

Intermittent exercise is acceptable to maintain the basic fitness of young and healthy dogs. When exercise has specific therapeutic or physical goals, however, it should be performed daily, with assiduity. Exercise may be fragmented into short sessions performed several times daily in patients with impaired mobility. For example, obese or old, arthritic dogs should ideally be exercised several times each day because exercise supports weight loss and helps maintain their mobility.

Little is known about the optimal duration of an exercise program. Seemingly, the maintenance of a basic fitness level does not require much exercise in dogs. Conditioning dogs, however, requires repetitive exercises lasting more than 10 minutes each time. Exercise sessions, as a consequence, generally last more than 10 minutes and often last 20 to 40 minutes. Dogs should show no sign of loss of performance (i.e., a lack of ability to continue to walk or an overt lameness) during the session. A loss of performance indicates that the duration or the intensity of an exercise session is excessive. The frequency or duration of an exercise session should be tailored to the owner's schedule. For people with tight schedules, exercise sessions can be shortened and their intensity may be increased. For example, jogging or training on an agility course for 15 minutes may be equivalent to walking for 25 minutes.

The Benefits of Exercising Dogs

Exercise maintains or increases cardiovascular and muscular fitness. While physical inactivity is a known risk factor for cardiovascular disease in humans, little is known about the effects of lack of physical activity on dogs' health. Furthermore, the exercise required for dogs to maintain their fitness level is not known. It seems logical, however, to think that fit dogs stay more active, mobile, and agile and therefore are less likely to become overweight and injure themselves. Dogs with limited mobility due to old age, chronic diseases, or injuries benefit from an exercise program aimed at increasing their fitness level. As an added benefit, dog walking appears to lead to a physically active lifestyle for dog owners.[2]

Physical inactivity is a known risk factor for obesity in humans, and it appears to be a risk factor for obesity in dogs as well. The risk of obesity decreases as physical activity increases in dogs.[3] Weight gain is the result of an imbalance between energy intake and energy expenditure, and exercise has a direct impact on energy expenditure.[4]

Exercise also influences energy intake (appetite). Energy intake increases in lean subjects with moderate to intense physical activity, allowing these subjects to maintain their body weight.[5] Moderate to intense physical activity does not appear to affect the energy intake of obese subjects. Importantly, energy intake does not decrease in subjects lacking physical activity. Decreased activity without a concurrent decrease in energy intake leads to weight gain. In the short term, this gain can be reversed by initiating physical activity (less than one hour/day).[5] Canine activity programs, including walking for 15 to 30 minutes or swimming for five to 15 minutes, have been proposed,[4] but there is no scientific data supporting a specific amount of activity for optimal weight loss in dogs.

Overweight dogs are unlikely to lose weight if their weight loss program solely rests on an increase in their exercise level. Dietary adjustments are required for weight loss. Overweight dogs are less mobile than dogs of normal weight and have a shorter life span. In a lifelong study of overweight and non-overweight Labrador Retrievers, the overweight dogs lived 18 months less than their non-overweight siblings. The key factor in the loss of longevity appeared to be the loss of mobility that occurred because of the presence of osteoarthritis in multiple joints in the thoracic and pelvic limbs combined with the added weight.[6] A combined owner-dog weight loss program led to improved participation for dogs enrolled in the program.[7]

Exercise strengthens both the limbs and the back and abdomen (i.e., the core). This increase in strength is particularly important in large and giant dog breeds because it protects them from a loss of mobility. Limb strength is achieved by performing repetitive exercises for more than 10 minutes. Core strength is possibly important in chondrodystrophic dogs (i.e., Basset Hounds, Dachshunds, etc.) because of their disproportionately short legs. Core strengthening is achieved by walking on irregular surfaces, walking on trails, or swimming. In a study of 48 Wirehaired Dachshunds, exercise (moderate stair climbing) and "duration of exercise" had moderate protective values with regard to intervertebral disk herniation.[8]

Exercise increases proprioception and balance. Weight-shifting exercises (i.e., walking on a soft or irregular surface or in water) stimulate proprioception. This has been most clearly documented in older people, in whom exercise protects mobility. Exercise also may be used to stretch joints. Walking uphill, for example, leads to a slight increase in hip joint extension compared to walking on a flat surface.[9]

The Risks for Exercising Dogs

Exercise carries inherent risks, including the risk of physical injury. Injury may occur because a dog is hit by a motor vehicle, hits a stationary object (i.e., fence post, tree, etc.), or slips. Dogs could also get lost during an exercise session. Exercise should be done with great caution when the ground is slippery (i.e., when exercising on ice, wet grass). The risk of a traumatic incident or loss appears greatly minimized when dogs are properly socialized and supervised.

There is a risk associated with having dogs play together particularly in dog parks where dogs of various sizes run together in groups. Several steps should be implemented to minimize the risks of injuries when dogs play together: the dogs should be of similar size, weight, and fitness level. Injuries are more likely when a less fit dog attempts to play with well conditioned dogs. Ideally the field of play should be free of obstacles, and the ground should provide good traction.

Dogs with undiagnosed or asymptomatic orthopedic problems may exhibit signs of lameness after exercise. These dogs may have osteoarthritis—secondary to hip or elbow dysplasia, for example—or a patellar luxation, a partial tear to a cranial cruciate ligament, or another problem. These orthopedic problems are very unlikely to be the result of exercise. Rather, the clinical signs may indicate a flare-up or an increase in the severity of the disease. In most cases, a period of rest followed by a return to low-impact exercises is sufficient to control the flare-up.

The Cost and Demands of Exercising Dogs

The cost and demands of exercise should be taken into account when discussing exercise in general and when designing a specific exercise program. The following logistical and financial principles apply to exercise:

1. Exercise is only possible for dogs that are willing and able to do it.
2. Exercising a dog always represents a time commitment for an owner.
3. Clinicians should always favor the exercise program that maximizes the owner's involvement (meaning that dogs should be exercised by their owners, unless there is a clear contraindication for owner involvement).
4. Exercise should be performed in a veterinary hospital when the dog is being trained to exercise, when the owner is being trained to exercise her dog, or when the exercise can only be done in that setting (e.g., when a dog is exercise-intolerant on land but exercises successfully in a swimming pool or an underwater treadmill). Over time, as the dog becomes better trained (and fitter) and the owner becomes better versed in overseeing exercise, the responsibility of exercising the dog should be transferred to the owner.

Because every owner brings a unique set of circumstances, the exercise program should be suited to that individual. For instance, how mobile is the owner? How enthusiastic and motivated is he about a lifelong exercise program? What goals does he have in mind? How socialized and malleable is the dog? How impaired is the dog (i.e., how critical is the exercise program)? Does the owner live in an urban, suburban, or rural environment?

The time involved in exercising a dog should be taken into account when making exercise recommendations. How much time will the owner dedicate to exercising her dog? If exercise cannot be done at home or from home, how much time will be spent traveling to and from the exercise location? Will the owner's availability fluctuate? How should the exercise program be adapted to fit her schedule?

Exercise programs should be planned with the long term in mind. The technician or clinician should ask himself, "What is the simplest exercise program that can achieve the goals set by the owners? Will this exercise program be sustainable over the long term? What will the yearly cost of the exercise program be? Should the owner invest in exercise equipment to be used at home (i.e., a land treadmill)?" Sporting activities often constitute a good form of exercise (as long as they are not excessively strenuous, such as flyball or long jump). Their cost is usually moderate and may be more sustainable than a home-based exercise program, because of the social network associated with the activity. Sporting activities require varying amount of strength, fitness, agility, and obedience. They may or may not be strenuous. Tracking, for example, is a low-impact activity that can be done by dogs with suboptimal physical fitness.

Exercise Misconceptions

There are several misconceptions regarding exercise among companion animal owners and clinicians. They originate from the fact that controlled, repetitive activity is a relatively new concept in companion animal medicine. In the past (and in the present, for some) the paradigm was that exercising always meant the equivalent of unbridled, uncontrolled freedom for dogs (Table 6.2). That is far from reality. The current paradigm is that exercise in a unique opportunity to provide controlled activity to companion animals. The key misconceptions regarding exercise are listed below.

Exercise is Detrimental to Overweight and Arthritic Dogs
The research performed in humans clearly supports the fact that exercise is beneficial to overweight patients and those with osteoarthritis.[10–13]

Exercise is Always Traumatic
Exercise is considered an automatic source of trauma by some clinicians. That concept is used to make the erroneous recommendation of decreasing exercise in overweight or arthritic dogs. Exercise is not always traumatic. While uncontrolled exercise periods may be trau-

Table 6.2. Ten fundamental rules of exercise in dog.

1. Exercise is beneficial to all dogs, even obese and arthritic dogs; it makes them stronger and fitter.
2. Exercise is not always traumatic. In fact, exercise programs rarely involve traumatic activities.
3. The best form of exercise in dogs is to take a long walk. Walks can vary greatly, depending on their speed, duration, slopes, and surfaces.
4. Retrieving a ball, a stick, or a flying disc is not a good form of exercise for dogs, particularly for large, heavyset dogs such as Labrador Retrievers. They are at risk of orthopedic injuries, and retrieving has little positive impact on their cardiovascular and muscle fitness.
5. Exercise programs, just like weight loss programs, are specifically tailored to dogs based on their profile and the expectations of their owners. To be sustained over a long period of time, exercises must be comfortable, fun, and convenient.
6. Exercises may be selected to achieve specific goals, including maintaining or increasing fitness, increasing limb and core strength, losing weight, alleviating osteoarthritis pain, stretching joints, and increasing balance and proprioception.
7. The successful implementation of an exercise program first requires that the dog learn to perform specific exercises, and then requires that the owner learn how to exercise his dog.
8. A veterinary technician or a veterinarian familiar with the patient may oversee the implementation and management of exercise programs. A fee schedule may be developed for this important service.
9. Aquatic exercises, including walking on an underwater treadmill and swimming under supervision, may be the only type of exercise for patients with compromised mobility because of excess weight or orthopedic diseases.
10. Exercise modifications do not greatly influence dogs' weight. Nutritional intervention is required for weight optimization.

matic, controlled exercises, such as leash walks (Figure 6.1) or swims, are not traumatic.

Retrieving is a Beneficial Form of Exercise

Subjectively, retrieving a ball or flying disc has little positive impact on the health of dogs because it is most often performed for a brief period of time (less than five minutes). In addition, retrieving may lead to orthopedic injuries associated with rapid acceleration and deceleration and falls.[10] Sustained low-impact exercises appear much safer and more beneficial than retrieving.

Dogs Get Their Exercise When They Are Left Outdoors, Unsupervised

Dog owners often count periods of unsupervised freedom (being outdoors in a fenced-in backyard, for example) as an exercise period. While the behavior of dogs is highly variable, many dogs exercise minimally (and sleep a lot) when left outdoors unsupervised. As a general rule, owners appear to overestimate the activity level of their dogs.[11]

Dogs Naturally Know How to Exercise

Many dogs are not trained to walk at a regular speed for sustained periods of time. Quite a few are not leash trained. Some misbehave. Some are not particularly fond of exercise. Others have physical limitations that complicate their exercise periods.

Owners Naturally Know How to Exercise their Dogs

Many owners are under the impression that dogs naturally fulfill their exercise needs (see misconceptions above) or have little training when it comes to exercising their dogs. They do not know how to train their dogs to perform specific exercises or how to recognize that an exercise is excessive or inappropriate. Most owners need to be taught how to exercise their dogs.

Exercise Options

Playing

Playing is a natural activity that involves running, changing direction, and jumping. Dogs can play with each other or with people. When playing with other dogs, dogs should ideally play with dogs with similar profiles (age, size, personality) to minimize the risk of injury. Playing often is an intense and strenuous form of exercise and its lack of predictability makes it a somewhat risky form of exercise that is not ideally suited to overweight dogs or those with pre-existing orthopedic problems.

Fetching

Fetching is a very popular form of activity in the general public. In a survey of exercise patterns for medium, large, or giant dogs, fetching was performed by more than half of the dogs and was the second most common form of activity behind walking (65%).[11] Fetching may involve a flying disc, a ball, or a piece of wood. Dogs retrieving hard objects such as branches are at risk of facial and oral injuries.[10]

Walking

Walking is the most popular form of exercise (Figure 6.1). Walking can be performed off leash or on a fixed or retractable leash. It may be done in most urban, suburban, or rural environments, as well as on most surfaces: concrete, asphalt, grass, dirt/gravel, mulch, sand, snow, etc. While walking is an extremely safe form of exercise, its risks include

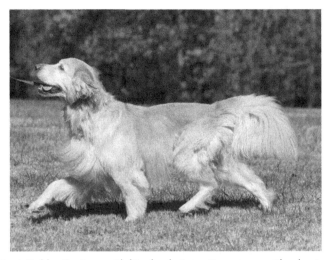

Figure 6.1. A Golden Retriever with hip dysplasia trotting on grass. The dog is well trained. He is controlled by a neck leash but he does not pull on the leash. His posture, facial expression, and tail carriage suggest that he is comfortable and enjoying the exercise. He has hip dysplasia that was diagnosed one year before, and is managed conservatively, primarily with daily exercise sessions. This illustration was made at the Animal Rehabilitation and Wellness Hospital in Raleigh, NC, and was made possible by Novartis Animal Health, Greensboro, NC.

motor vehicle accidents (particularly when off leash or with retractable leashes) and injuries to footpads that may be caused by grass awns, sand spurs, oyster shells, etc.[12] Asphalt may be too hot for dogs to walk on in hot weather conditions.

Walking is accessible and beneficial to all types of dogs: young and old, fit and unfit, healthy and injured. Its benefits include socializing and developing obedience in young dogs, enhancing cardiovascular and muscle fitness (limb strength, core strength), promoting limb use, and losing weight. The speed, duration, surface, slope, and surroundings of the walk should be adapted to the patient's personality, physical health, and preferences. Walking may be done on a treadmill (Figure 6.2) or in an underwater treadmill (Figure 6.3) as part of a therapeutic or conditioning program or when it is impossible to exercise outdoors.

Locomotion assistance may be offered to dogs with impaired mobility. Such assistance may help weak, painful, obese, or unfit dogs start an exercise program. As the exercise program progresses, the ambulation assistance may consist of a chest harness (Figure 6.4), a pelvic limb harness made of nylon or neoprene (Figure 6.5), an ambulation cart, a hoist, or ambulation in water. The buoyancy provided by having water up to the hip region greatly facilitates stance and walk. The force placed on limbs decreases by approximately two-thirds when dog are immersed to their greater trochanter. The ambulation

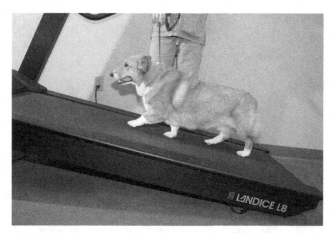

Figure 6.2. A dog engaged in a weight maintenance and fitness program trotting uphill on a treadmill. The dog lost 8 kg (17 pounds) during the program. A treadmill is a convenient and effective exercise method for dogs because duration, speed, slope, and temperature are easily controlled. This illustration was made at the Animal Rehabilitation and Wellness Hospital in Raleigh, NC, and was made possible by Novartis Animal Health, Greensboro, NC.

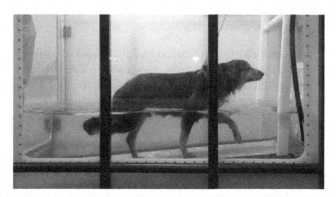

Figure 6.3. A dog trotting on an immersed treadmill. The treadmill is sloped upward by approximately 8°. Buoyancy facilitates locomotion by decreasing the forces that the dog must generate to support his own weight. On the other hand, the cohesion of water molecules increases the forces that the dog must generate to move forward on the treadmill. This illustration was made at the Animal Rehabilitation and Wellness Hospital in Raleigh, NC, and was made possible by Novartis Animal Health, Greensboro, NC.

assistance provided by underwater treadmills is comfortable and therefore does not interfere with the duration of an exercise session (Figure 6.3). By comparison, the ambulation assistance provided by lifting devices (slings, carts) tends to be much less comfortable and the devices often interfere with the quality and duration of an exercise session. Ambulation carts may be used to promote the mobility of severely

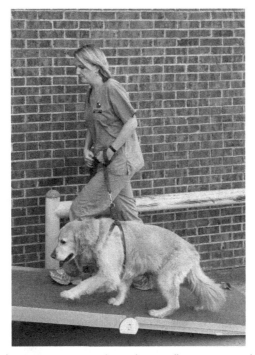

Figure 6.4. The dog in Figure 6.1 is shown here walking up a metal ramp covered with non-skid rubber. Ramps, slopes, and steps may be climbed repeatedly to strengthen pelvic limbs. This is particularly useful if walking up and down stairs is part of the dog's daily functional activities. The dog is controlled by a chest harness, which may be used for control and to provide locomotion assistance. This illustration was made at the Animal Rehabilitation and Wellness Hospital in Raleigh, NC, and was made possible by Novartis Animal Health, Greensboro, NC.

impaired dogs. See the list of resources for ambulation assistance devices at the end of this chapter.

Static Exercises

Static exercises are performed in one location, usually while the dog is standing on the ground, a wobble or balance board (Figure 6.6), or an exercise ball. Changing position, such as moving from a sitting to a standing position is another static exercise. These exercises usually are performed in the early postoperative period or to address limb disuse (a long-standing reluctance to use a limb because of a chronic orthopedic problem).[13] The benefits of static exercises include limb and core strengthening for weak and extremely unfit patients (neurologic patients with impaired motor function, overweight geriatric patients), promoting limb use through forced weight-shifting, stimulating proprioceptive inputs, and training balance.

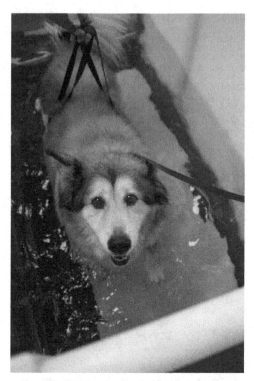

Figure 6.5. A dog with severe hip osteoarthritis exercising in an underwater treadmill. The dog's weight is supported by the water and by a nylon sling. The dog is more relaxed and he exercises much more effectively in the underwater treadmill than on land. This illustration was made at the Animal Rehabilitation and Wellness Hospital in Raleigh, NC, and was made possible by Novartis Animal Health, Greensboro, NC.

Mixed Dynamic Exercises

Mixed dynamic exercises may be therapeutic (i.e., address a specific medical problem), used to stretch or promote overall fitness (limb strength, core strength) or be part of sporting activities (agility, flyball, flying discs, obedience, etc.). Mixed exercises may be performed in suburban environments, for example by climbing on and off a curb or going around trees. Cavaletti rails (a handful of horizontal bars placed a few feet apart) are commonly used as a mixed exercise to promote weight shifting, stretch joints (in flexion), and stimulate proprioception (Figure 6.7).

Swimming

Swimming is a popular form of exercise for dogs. It may take place in a natural body of water (pond, lake, river, ocean), a swimming pool, or a swim tank. Swimming is used for conditioning purposes and, albeit

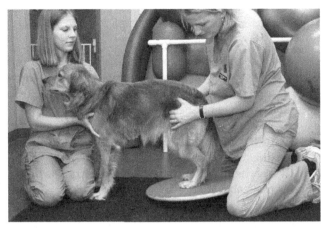

Figure 6.6. A dog exercising on a wobble board. His pelvic limbs straddle the center of the board, and once the clinician removes her hands the dog keeps the board balanced for a period of time. Wobble boards stimulate proprioception and balance. Balancing on a wobble board exercises core muscles of the abdomen and back. This illustration was made at the Animal Rehabilitation and Wellness Hospital in Raleigh, NC, and was made possible by Novartis Animal Health, Greensboro, NC.

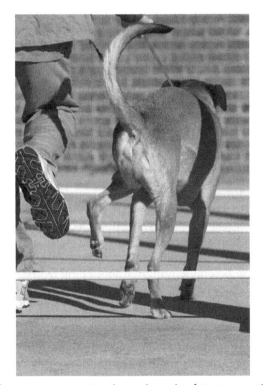

Figure 6.7. A dog trotting across Cavaletti rails made of PVC pipes. The rails are placed approximately at the level of the dog's talo-crural joints. Clearing the rails increases flexion of the stifle joint, compared to walking on a flat surface. Walking across Cavaletti rails may be used to promote limb use and to gently stretch the stifle joint in flexion. This illustration was made at the Animal Rehabilitation and Wellness Hospital in Raleigh, NC, and was made possible by Novartis Animal Health, Greensboro, NC.

less frequently, for therapeutic purposes.[14] The benefits of swimming include increasing cardiovascular and muscle fitness, increasing core strength, and exercising without bearing weight (for patients with joint pain exacerbated by weight-bearing). Swimming may range widely in intensity depending on the personality of the dog and whether or not a therapist is in the pool with the dog. Also, the use of pelvic limbs varies among dogs; some use all four limbs when they swim, whereas others mostly use their forelimbs and keep their pelvic limbs flexed and tucked under their abdomen.

Planning an Exercise Program

The dog's profile should be taken into account when planning an exercise program. Some dogs naturally like physical activity, and others don't. Young dogs are naturally more active than older dogs. Large dogs, as a general rule, are naturally more active than small dogs, but that rule has numerous exceptions. The following questions should be asked when planning an exercise program:

What Are the Overall Goals for This Dog?

Goals may include maintaining or increasing fitness,[1] strengthening the core and limbs, losing weight, increasing the use of a limb, stretching, and increasing balance and proprioception.

How Much Exercise and What Exercises Should Be Used to Achieve These Goals?

Increasing endurance requires a minimum of 10 minutes of sustained repetitive muscular activity. At least three exercise sessions/week are most likely necessary to positively impact a dog's cardiovascular fitness. Caloric expenditure is increased during exercise and for several hours afterward. Exercise programs aimed at increasing fitness or endurance are designed to be challenging without being overwhelming.

Are the Proposed Exercises Safe for This Particular Dog?

High-intensity exercises should be avoided in patients with weak (unstable) joints. Jumping or slipping is inherently riskier for large and heavy dogs compared to small and light dogs. Playing with other dogs is better suited to dogs with thicker bones and tendons than to dogs with thin bones and tendons. That is the rationale for the use of Lurchers (crossbred sighthounds that have relatively thick bones and tendons) for the training of young racing Greyhounds. Falls should be avoided in patients with impaired balance and in dogs from large and giant breeds.

Is the Dog Comfortable With all Aspects of the Proposed Exercise Program?

Clinicians should not assume that dogs will naturally perform all types of exercise and that a brief description of an exercise will suffice for an owner to properly supervise his dog. Ideally, exercises should initally be supervised by the technician or clinician, who should assess whether the dog is willing and able to engage in these specific exercises. Next, the clinician should train the dog during a few exercise sessions, and finally she should train the owner to exercise the dog.

It is not unusual to need a "break in" or socialization period when initiating an exercise program. This may include teaching the dog to exercise while being controlled by a neck collar or a chest harness and a leash. Owners can only successfully exercise their dogs when they accurately assess the comfort level and proper gait of their dogs. For many owners, this may require specific training that involves both the owner and therapist jointly exercising a dog.

Where and When Should Dogs Exercise?

The location and time of exercise should be discussed with the owner to make sure that it is practical, safe, and effective.

How Will the Exercise Program Evolve Over Time?

The re-evaluation schedule should be discussed. Will some exercise sessions occur at the clinic? How rapidly will the dog reach the weight and fitness goals? Weight loss and conditioning programs routinely last 10 to 20 weeks.

Once these fundamental questions are addressed, a clinician should propose an exercise program to the owner. The program should be convenient, stimulating, safe, and adapted to the dog's profile. The owner's motivation should be sustained through regular communication with the staff overseeing the exercise program. It may be helpful for the owner to keep an exercise log that is reviewed periodically by the technician or clinician. Often, the exercise program is paired with a nutrition program and progress of both programs are simultaneously evaluated at regular intervals, perhaps monthly.

In the author's experience, exercise programs are more likely to succeed when they are initiated under the supervision of a trained staff member who trains the dog and then teaches the owner to exercise her dog. The most fundamental (and popular)[11] exercise program consists of regular leash walks. Over time, the walks may increase in duration, intensity (speed, slopes), or frequency. Leash walks are simple, convenient, safe, and effective. Beyond leash walks, healthy, energetic dogs whose owners are inclined to engage in sporting activities may perform tracking, agility, herding, obedience, etc. Dogs that are too weak, unfit, or unruly to go on leash walks should be exercised in the clinic initially, with a later transition to home-based exercise programs. Clinic-based exercises should be the simplest exercise programs that will help owners reach their goals. Aquatic exercises may be a consideration for weak and unfit dogs, particularly walking in an underwater treadmill. Underwater treadmills allow dogs to have brief periods of assisted ambulation separated by periods of rest. Early on, dogs may only be able to walk for one or two minutes and may need to rest for five minutes between walking periods. The exercise-to-rest ratio usually increases rapidly when dogs exercise regularly, such as twice weekly or more.

Swimming may be considered for dogs with impaired limb use or impaired locomotion. However, unlike underwater treadmills, it is challenging to alternate periods of rest and periods of exercise in a swim tank. That may be achievable if the therapist is in the swim tank with the dog and holds the dog calmly between swimming periods. Overall, however, successful exercise in locomotion-impaired dogs is easier to achieve in an underwater treadmill than in a swim tank. Furthermore, whereas dogs reliably use their pelvic limbs when they walk in an underwater treadmill, pelvic limb use is not very predictable when dogs swim.

Other forms of exercise may be included in an exercise program. Often owners seek variety and challenges beyond leash walks or swimming, or they wish to achieve specific goals, including promoting the use of a limb that is not used properly at a walk, trot, or while swimming; stretching joints that have limited motion; or promoting balance and proprioception. Promoting limb use is an important part of exercise programs in patients with chronic orthopedic problems who have fallen into a limb disuse situation. Limb disuse may be associated with loss of muscle mass (and bone mass), loss of joint motion because of periarticular fibrosis, local amplification of noxious sensory stimuli, and changes in body posture. Locomotion on soft and unsteady surfaces as well as on dry and underwater treadmills promotes limb use in these patients.

Exercise may be used to stretch joints. From a scientific perspective, little is known about the relative benefits of manual stretching and stretching through exercise in dogs with limited joint motion. From a practical perspective, manual stretching is a difficult task for owners who may not have the discipline to do it regularly (i.e., two to three times daily) and who may be afraid to hurt their dogs. In the author's experience, stretching through exercise is therefore more likely to be achievable and to lead to a positive outcome.

Stretching exercises include static exercises such as standing on an exercise ball or active exercises such as walking over Cavaletti rails or walking with a hypermetric gait in an underwater treadmill filled with

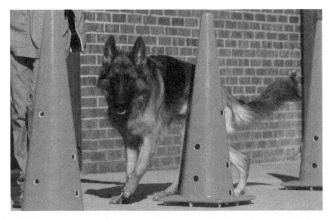

Figure 6.8. A dog zigzagging between traffic cones. The handler controls the path followed by the dog and keeps that path unpredictable. The rapid changes in direction stimulate proper weight distribution among limbs. This may be used to promote limb use in patients with disuse. Rapid changes in direction also strengthen core muscles and train balance. This illustration was made at the Animal Rehabilitation and Wellness Hospital in Raleigh, NC, and was made possible by Novartis Animal Health, Greensboro, NC.

water up to the stifle joint. It is much easier to stretch joints in flexion than in extension through active exercises (Figure 6.7). Static exercises and dancing backwards may be used to stretch joints in extension.[9] An increase in hip extension, albeit quite small, also occurs when dogs are walking uphill, compared to walking on flat surfaces.[9]

Promoting balance and proprioception often is indicated in the management of patients recovering from a herniated intervertebral disc or patients with progressive neuropathies such as degenerative myelopathy (Figure 6.8). Promoting balance and proprioception is also a consideration when exercising high-performance dogs (agility dogs, field trial dogs, flyball dogs, etc.) and when exercising geriatric patients.

Assessing and Adjusting Exercise Programs

Because little is known about the ideal amount of exercise in dogs, most exercise programs initially include a subjective amount of exercise that fits the dog's and owner's profiles. The average program includes 20 to 30 minutes of daily physical activity. Assessing the response to that initial program is critical to optimizing the activity of specific patients.

The assessment of an exercise program includes a review of the type, intensity, duration, and frequency of exercises. When a dog is exercised at home, the owner should record the exercise information, and when enrolled in a clinic-based exercise program, a technician records that information. The duration of exercise is easily recorded, usually in minutes. Because exercise may not be constant, for example when a dog takes a walk and stops to sniff or rest, it may be optimal to record both the overall duration of an exercise session and the duration of the activity or the distance covered during that period of time.

The intensity is the speed at which an exercise is performed. For example, what gait is the dog using when taking a walk (the walk, pace, or trot)? If a dog exercises on a treadmill, what is the speed of the treadmill? The frequency of exercise is easily recorded: How many times a week is the dog exercising? Other exercise parameters to record include the slopes of the ground where the dog exercises, the ground surfaces, and the time of the day. Finally, the performance of the dog during exercise and his/her comfort afterward should be recorded.

A review of the exercise log greatly facilitates the assessment of the exercise program. It also helps the technician or clinician and owner identify patterns such as which activity is best tolerated and which time of day is best for exercise. The patient's progress should be assessed objectively and recorded. Is the exercise program progressing as intended? Are there signs of orthopedic problems or fatigue, suggesting that the program is too intense? Is the owner's motivation maintained? Are there objective signs of improved fitness, strength, or body condition? The exercise program should be adjusted based on the results of that assessment. The intensity and duration of exercise sessions should be modified, some activities may be discontinued, and new activities may be introduced.

The re-evaluation schedule of patients enrolled in exercise programs should be based the severity of their initial problems. An obese dog that is reluctant to exercise should be re-evaluated after a week or two. A young, overweight dog without orthopedic problems may be re-evaluated after a month or two. A technician may oversee the re-evaluation, provided that the exercise program is progressing well and that the dog is showing no signs of lameness or exercise intolerance. The exercise program should be modified based on the results of the re-evaluation. The overall activity level may be increased in dogs that do not appear to be challenged by their current program. On the other hand, the overall activity level should be decreased in dogs that struggle at their current activity level.

Exercising Dogs With Medical Conditions

Obesity

Obese dogs may or may not have chronic orthopedic problems. The exercise considerations for obese dogs with osteoarthritis are described below. Obese dogs with healthy limbs are clear candidate for exercise programs because the increased caloric expenditure resulting from exercise will assist them in their ongoing weight loss program and their future weight maintenance program.

Several factors are considered when their exercise program is designed: cardiovascular and muscle fitness level, potential heat intolerance, and lack of agility. Because locomotion is more strenuous for obese dogs, their exercise sessions may have to be short, particularly when exercising in hot weather. To offset this, the frequency of exercise can be increased to two or three daily sessions. As dogs lose weight, the duration and intensity of their exercise sessions should increase and their frequency may decrease. Aquatic exercises are very suited to obese dogs that are reluctant to walk because the buoyancy of the water offsets their excess weight. For some obese dogs, aquatic exercises are the only feasible exercises.

Because obese dogs are at increased risk of orthopedic injuries, strenuous exercises, including those with rapid acceleration, deceleration, sudden changes in direction, jumping, slipping, or falling, should be avoided. These exercises include playing with other dogs outdoors, retrieving, and catching flying discs and balls. Retrieving an object floating in water is safe.

Osteoarthritis

By some estimates, approximately 20% of adult dogs have osteoarthritis (OA). Many arthritic dogs also are overweight, in part because they spontaneously limit their activity or because their owner or veterinarian decided to limit the dogs' activity. Exercise is clearly beneficial to humans with OA; people with OA can pursue a high level of physical activity, provided that activity is not painful and does not predispose to trauma.[15] The benefits of exercises with regard to OA pain and function are only maintained if exercise is performed regularly. In humans, exercise should be performed one to three times/week. Professional assistance can be helpful in improving initial compliance and perseverance. Exercise leads to an immediate moderate decrease in pain and an immediate mild improvement in function.[1] By extension, it appears logical to consider setting up and sustaining exercise programs for arthritic dogs so they can stay fit and strong. In fact, OA often is discovered later in life in very active dogs compared to sedentary dogs, because the signs of OA tend to be less obvious in active dogs compared to sedentary dogs.

Dogs with OA have variable clinical signs that increase over a lifetime. Many are asymptomatic during the first few years of life; afterwards, dogs with OA tend to have intermittent flare-ups. Over time, flare-ups become more severe, more common, and harder to control. Later, the clinical signs are constant and dogs may become exercise intolerant (i.e., unwilling to go on walks). As they age, dogs with severe OA may lose the ability to walk.

Asymptomatic dogs with OA may exercise like all other dogs. The activity of dogs with OA should be planned and discussed with their owners. It should be adapted to fit their needs (based on their energy level and limitations) and to fit the owners' expectations. Activities that lead to OA flare-ups should be avoided. On the other hand, activities that do not lead to clinical signs of OA, such as lameness, difficulty climbing or going down steps, vocalization, changes in demeanor, and restlessness at night, should be promoted. The healthiest forms of activity for dogs with OA are low-impact, repetitive exercises such as leash walks. High-impact exercises, those that require jumping, repeated accelerations and decelerations, or changes in direction, are unlikely to be beneficial to dogs with OA and may trigger OA flare-ups. Spontaneous activity, such as being left unsupervised in a fenced-in backyard, also is unlikely to be beneficial to dogs with OA because most dogs do not move for sustained periods of time when left unsupervised. Clinicians generally recommend rest during OA flare-ups, even though there is no scientific evidence in humans that supports stopping exercise during flare-ups.[15] For patients between OA flare-ups, pain relief may be enhanced by therapeutic exercises that strengthen muscles, improve posture, and increase proprioception. Clinical trials in humans with knee or hip OA have clearly documented that exercises have unique benefits for OA patients.[16] Strengthening exercises also have proven benefits in dogs recovering from cranial cruciate ligament stabilization.[17]

It is very important to assess and manage pain in OA patients because pain may interfere with the their willingness to exercise regularly. Although many medications have been proposed in the management of OA in dogs, most medications lack scientific (evidence-based) proof of efficacy. The exception is nonsteroidal anti-inflammatory drugs, which are clearly efficacious for the management of signs of OA.[18] Beyond that, several nutritional strategies have demonstrated promising positive results for managing signs of OA.[23] Icing superficial arthritic joints many be of benefit in dogs with OA that have flare-ups or that have just completed an exercise session. Pain also can be minimized by cautiously selecting the type, time, and surfaces for the exercises and by avoiding excessively strenuous or long periods of exercise (i.e., avoiding the weekend warrior syndrome).

Older dogs with OA may lose the ability to function independently. Classically, mobility disorders include difficulty getting up, the reluctance to climb or walk down stairs, difficulty walking on slippery surfaces (i.e., hardwood floors, tiles), sitting in the middle of a leash walk, and the lack of ability to run or trot. Ambulation assistance, which includes the use of ramps, steps, chest harnesses, slings, and ambulation carts, may be used to help these dogs (see list of resources at the end of this chapter). An underwater treadmill can provide ambulation assistance during therapeutic exercises. The type and intensity of ambulation assistance should be proportionate to the severity of the disease.

Table 6.3. Factors influencing the recovery rate after injury or surgery in dogs.

Factor	Rapid recovery	Slow recovery
Mobility	Medium size	Large or giant size
	Normal weight	Overweight or obese
	Proper fitness	Loss of physical conditioning
Strength	Proper muscle mass	Loss of muscle mass
		Neurologic disease
Joint motion	Unrestricted, pain-free range	Limited (swelling, fibrosis, contractures)
Pain	Controlled	Uncontrolled
Chronicity	Recent problems	Chronic problems
	Single surgery	Repeated surgeries

Orthopedic Surgery

Exercise programs also are important in dogs recovering from orthopedic surgical procedures. The exercise program should take into account the strength of the surgical repair and the patient's stage of recovery. Exercise programs after surgery are aimed primarily at avoiding long-term limb disuse and the associated loss of range of motion (resulting most often from excessive periarticular fibrosis), loss of muscle mass, and changes in body posture. Postoperative exercise programs are also aimed at protecting or recovering limb strength (muscle mass).

Gentle weight shifting and stretching exercises are used in the early postoperative period.[13] Strengthening exercises are used later. The rhythm of therapy should be adapted to the patient. The importance of rest during recovery cannot be overemphasized. Dogs recovering from surgery should be given ample time to sleep in the first couple of postoperative days. To optimize their rest, therapy sessions may be combined with walks outside for urination and defecation and with feeding. In overactive patients, those with short attention span (puppies), and weak patients, therapy sessions should be shorter and occur more often than in calmer patients. Therapy should follow a logical progression, the rate of which depends on the anticipated recovery rate of each patient. Due to the wide variability in patients' cardiovascular and muscle fitness levels, personality, socialization, pain threshold, joint disease, and surgical trauma, recovery rates in patients vary widely (Table 6.3).

Recovery rates are more rapid in patients with good basic mobility and proper muscle mass. For example, one would anticipate more rapid limb use after cranial cruciate ligament stabilization using tibial plateau leveling than extracapsular stabilization. Subjectively, that may result from the fact that the stifle joint feels more comfortable after plateau leveling than after extracapsular stabilization. In the long term, however, this difference may not lead to functional differences between dogs undergoing these two surgical procedures.[19] The length, frequency, and intensity of leash walks should be adapted to the intrinsic willingness and ability to use the limb rather than an abstract decision based on theoretical recommendations. For some patients, a two-minute-long walk 10 days after surgery is perfectly acceptable. The clinician in charge of the dog's recovery should ensure that patients reach specific progress milestones within certain time intervals, but should not have inflexible predetermined schedules for the specific dates and amount of activity during recovery.

For example, during recovery after stabilization of a cranial cruciate ligament rupture, one would expect edema to be eliminated by day three, limb use (weight-bearing at a stance and during walk) to be initiated by day five, weight-bearing at a trot to be initiated by day 14, stifle joint extension to be equal to preoperative stifle joint extension by day 28, and thigh muscle mass to be symmetrical by day 56. Patients who meet these milestones on time are likely to be well managed. Patients that miss these milestones may be dealing with particular challenges (Table 6.2) or may have complications. In this case, mechanical failure, limb disuse, loss of stifle joint motion, meniscal tear, and infection are the most common complications.

Resources for Ambulation Assistance Devices

Device	Manufacturer*	Website
Boots		
	Ruff Wear	www.ruffwear.com
	Thera-paw	www.therapaw.com
Orthoses including sleeves, braces		
	Dynasplint Systems	www.dynasplint.com
	K-9 Orthotics and Prosthetics Inc.	www.k-9orthotics.com
	OrthoVet	www.orthovet.com
Straps bands		
	Biko Physio Brace	www.biko.co.at
	DogLeggs	www.dogleggs.com
Slings		
	Total Support Harness	www.helpemup.com
	Walkabout Harnesses	www.walkaboutharnesses.com
Ambulation carts		
	Canine Wheelchair Project	web.mac.com/gbertocci
	Canine Wheels	www.caninewheels.com
	Doggon' Wheels	www.doggon.com
	Eddie's Wheels for Pets	www.eddieswheels.com
	K-9 carts	www.k-9carts.com
	Walkin' Wheels	www.walkinwheels.com

*Manufacturers may sell products in several categories. Each manufacturer is listed once.

References

1. Marcellin-Little DJ, Levine D, Taylor R. 2005. Rehabilitation and conditioning of sporting dogs. *Vet Clin North Am Small Anim Pract* 35:1427–1439, ix.

2. Ham SA, Epping J. 2006. Dog walking and physical activity in the United States. *Prev Chronic Dis* 3:A47.

3. Robertson ID. 2003. The association of exercise, diet and other factors with owner-perceived obesity in privately owned dogs from metropolitan Perth, WA. *Prev Vet Med* 58:75–83.

4. Roudebush P, Schoenherr WD, Delaney SJ. 2008. An evidence-based review of the use of therapeutic foods, owner education, exercise, and drugs for the management of obese and overweight pets. *J Am Vet Med Assoc* 233:717–725.

5. Melzer K, Kayser B, Saris WH, et al. 2005. Effects of physical activity on food intake. *Clin Nutr* 24:885–895.

6. Lawler DF, Evans RH, Larson BT, et al. 2005. Influence of lifetime food restriction on causes, time, and predictors of death in dogs. *J Am Vet Med Assoc* 226:225–231.

7. Kushner RF, Blatner DJ, Jewell DE, et al. 2006. The PPET study: People and pets exercising together. *Obesity (Silver Spring)* 14:1762–1770.

8. Jensen VF, Ersboll AK. 2000. Mechanical factors affecting the occurrence of intervertebral disc calcification in the dachshund—a population study. *J Vet Med A Physiol Pathol Clin Med* 47:283–296.

9. Weigel JP, Arnold G, Hicks DA, et al. 2005. Biomechanics of rehabilitation. *Vet Clin North Am Small Anim Pract* 35:1255–1285, vii.

10. Australian Veterinary Association Media Release. 2005. AVA warns: Sticks and stones can break dogs' bones. http://avacms.eseries.hengesystems.com.au/AM/Template.cfm?Section=2005_Media_Releases, December 19, 2005.

11. Slater MR, Robinson LE, Zoran DL, et al. 1995. Diet and exercise patterns in pet dogs. *J Am Vet Med Assoc* 207:186–190.

12. Brennan KE, Ihrke PJ. 1983. Grass awn migration in dogs and cats: A retrospective study of 182 cases. *J Am Vet Med Assoc* 182:1201–1204.

13. Marcellin-Little DJ, Freeman J. 2005. Rehabilitation after stifle joint surgery. *NAVC Clinician's Brief* 4:39–43.

14. Marsolais GS, McLean S, Derrick T, et al. 2003. Kinematic analysis of the hind limb during swimming and walking in healthy dogs and dogs with surgically corrected cranial cruciate ligament rupture. *J Am Vet Med Assoc* 222:739–743.

15. Vignon E, Valat JP, Rossignol M, et al. 2006. Osteoarthritis of the knee and hip and activity: A systematic international review and synthesis (OASIS). *Joint Bone Spine* 73:442–455.

16. O'Reilly SC, Muir KR, Doherty M. 1999. Effectiveness of home exercise on pain and disability from osteoarthritis of the knee: A randomised controlled trial. *Ann Rheum Dis* 58:15–19.

17. Monk ML, Preston CA, McGowan CM. 2006. Effects of early intensive post-operative physiotherapy on limb function after tibial plateau leveling osteotomy in dogs with deficiency of the cranial cruciate ligament. *J Am Vet Med Assoc* 228:725.
18. Aragon CL, Hofmeister EH, Budsberg SC. 2007. Systematic review of clinical trials of treatments for osteoarthritis in dogs. *J Am Vet Med Assoc* 230:514–521.
19. Cook JL, Luther JK, Beetem J, et al. 2010. Clinical comparison of a novel extracapsular stabilization procedure and tibial plateau leveling osteotomy for treatment of cranial cruciate ligament deficiency in dogs. *Vet Surg* 39:315–323.

Owner Education and Adherence

Kara Burns, MS, MEd, LVT, and Todd L. Towell, DVM, MS, DACVIM

The most prevalent form of malnutrition in North American pets is excessive intake of calories, which results in excess body fat.[1] It is estimated that 24% to 30% of dogs and cats presenting to small animal hospitals in North America are overweight or obese. For pets aged 5 to 12 years, the prevalence increases to 40%.[2] Dogs and cats evaluated for excess weight are typically divided into two categories: those weighing 10% to 19% more than the optimal weight for their breed are considered overweight; those weighing 20% or more above the optimum are considered obese.[3] An extra five pounds on a dog that should weigh 17 pounds or an extra three pounds on a cat whose target weight is 10 pounds is equivalent to an extra 50 pounds on a person whose weight should be 170 pounds (Figure 7.1).

As discussed in Chapter 1, overweight pets are at increased risk for many illnesses, including heart disease, respiratory problems, diabetes, and osteoarthritis.[3–5] These pets also are at risk for a shorter life span; studies have shown that lean pets may live one to two years longer than those that are overweight.[4] Moreover, obesity can complicate or exacerbate other disease conditions. Veterinary technicians can assist the veterinarian and health care team in diagnosing and managing excess body fat and in educating the pet owner about the detrimental effects of this condition.

Owning (or being owned by) a pet is quite different in this decade than in the past. Dogs and cats are now members of the family, considered by most as "four-legged children." It was not long ago that dogs

Practical Weight Management in Dogs and Cats, First Edition. Edited by Todd L. Towell.
© 2011 John Wiley and Sons, Inc. Published 2011 by John Wiley & Sons, Inc.

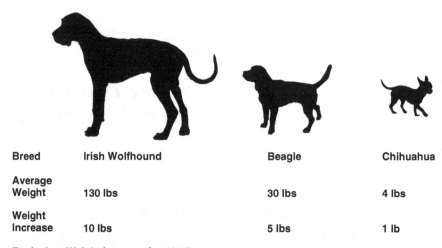

Breed	Irish Wolfhound	Beagle	Chihuahua
Average Weight	130 lbs	30 lbs	4 lbs
Weight Increase	10 lbs	5 lbs	1 lb

Equivalent Weight increase for 125-lb woman

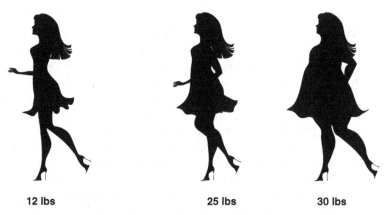

| 12 lbs | 25 lbs | 30 lbs |

Figure 7.1. Equivalent weight gains for people and various size pets. Images from Fotolia.com.

and cats had a "job" to do: dogs guarded the house or assisted with hunting, and cats were responsible for keeping the property clear of mice. Today, our pets listen to us but do not judge us, and make us smile and laugh. They bring us constant joy. Pet ownership has even been shown to have positive medical impacts on our health.

Pet owners have been shown to have lower blood pressure and cholesterol levels than those who do not own pets. Pet owners also have better odds of surviving a heart attack, have diminished chronic pain, and are less medicated, less lonely, and subsequently less depressed.[6] Studies have shown that the simple act of petting a companion animal decreases blood pressure and increases those "feel good" hormones. The same has been shown to be true for pets—as they are petted, their blood pressure drops and their hormones increase, leading to that same good feeling. The bond between people and their pets is truly a symbiotic relationship.

Key Point

Pet ownership is associated with improved health in people.

The Human-Animal Bond: What Goes Wrong?

Pets depend on us for health care, proper nutrition, and love to ensure good health and a long life. This is the human-animal bond—the unspoken love and devotion that people and pets share. However, the human-animal bond also can lead to pet obesity. It is undeniable that pet owners love their pets; unfortunately many owners "love" their pets to death. In a 2002 habits and practices study, pet owners were asked how they and other members of their household show affection toward each dog or cat.[7] Of more than 1,200 dog owners surveyed, 71% stated they showed affection by giving treats and 42% stated they showed affection by giving people food. Of 820 cat owners, 44% said they gave treats and 25% gave people food to their cat as a way of showing affection.[7] Owners believe that to show their pets love is to give them food, especially treats (Figure 7.2).

Obesity can well be declared an epidemic of people in the United States, with an estimated 127 million overweight adults. Over the past 25 years the prevalence of obesity in the U.S. has increased more than 40%.[8] Today, society is fast paced and most people are stressed and sedentary. The technological era has provided us with up-to-the-second information that we access from our desks or on our couches. The obesity epidemic is also perpetuated by the bigger is better mentality and the popularity of fast food. People eat more readily available yet less healthy foods, and exercise less. The bond humans feel with their pets often results in the passing of this lifestyle to their pets. Many

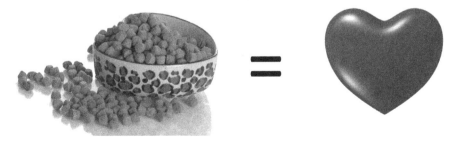

Figure 7.2. For many owners, food equals love. Images from Fotolia.com.

owners feel compelled to keep their pets' bowls full at all times and share their own food with their "four-legged children." Certainly, most dogs are thrilled to share dinner or dessert with their owner.

The fast pace of life in the new millennium also has resulted in the rise of two-income households, with all family members involved in a number of activities. This constant rushing behavior leads to unaccountability for certain household responsibilities, one of these being "Who feeds Fido and Fluffy?" This responsibility may be designated to one family member, but in the chaos of daily life another family member may also feed the pet, not realizing the pet had already been fed. Most pets readily accept a second helping without giving any indication that they have already eaten. Obviously, overfeeding on a regular basis results in the pet becoming overweight or obese.

Today, many people have a distorted view of portion sizes. It is no secret that portion sizes, as well as waistlines, in the U.S. are expanding. Restaurant meals, snack foods, and soft drinks have all gotten larger, with an emphasis on getting more food for the money. In fact, finding a 1oz. ounce bag of snack food or an 8oz. soft drink, which are the recommended single serving sizes, can be very difficult. Americans are surrounded by larger portion sizes at relatively low prices, which appeals to consumer's economic sensibilities. This distorted view of portion sizes often is applied to pets as well. It is common for owners to overestimate the volume of food that constitutes a meal for their pet. Although the health care team may provide clients with a specific nutritional recommendation, including type of food and amount to be fed, this recommendation may be misunderstood by the client.

For example, take a pet owner who is instructed to give one cup of food twice a day. If the health care team does not define "one cup," the pet owner may use the 32oz. "cup" he purchased at the convenience store (Figure 7.3). The veterinary technician assumes the client knows the recommendation is for one 8oz. cup but the client assumed "a cup" refers to the portion size he uses to refill his drinks. Although owners

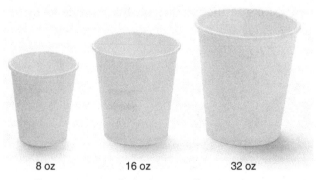

| 8 oz | 16 oz | 32 oz |

Figure 7.3. Not all cups are created equal. Images from Fotolia.com.

may believe they are being kind to their pets by being generous with portion sizes, the cost to their health may be higher than most people realize.

Studies show that people eat more when they are confronted with larger portion sizes. Early observational work suggests this also may be true for pets as well. Several studies have documented that neutered cats and dogs may lose the ability to self regulate intake. Therefore, that extra 24 oz. of food provided by the 32 oz. cup will quickly result in overconsumption of food and weight gain. No malice was intended by either party, but now the pet is gaining weight.

Weight Reduction Programs

As with humans, when a dog or cat takes in more energy (i.e., calories) than it expends, a positive energy balance results. The unused energy is stored by the body as fat. Pets become overweight or obese when they are in a positive energy balance for an extended period. Genetics, spaying or neutering, age, physical activity, and caloric composition of food are risk factors for positive energy balance, weight gain, and ultimately, obesity.[4,8] It is critical for the health care team to help clients understand these risk factors as part of treating or preventing obesity in their pets.

Designing a Weight Loss Program

Designing a successful weight reduction program is a multi-step process involving a specific feeding plan, careful patient monitoring, and good communication between the owner and the health care team (Figure 7.4). As previously mentioned, technicians should play a key role in the process by determining the pet's ideal weight and educating owners about the health risks associated with being overweight or obese. The health care team must effectively communicate to the owner the importance of weight loss and the owner must accept the team's recommendation. If one of these steps is missing, the program will fail.

Communication

Effective communication is essential for gaining commitment from the pet owner. Effective communication is best achieved through relationship centered care. In veterinary medicine, relationship centered care represents a joint venture between the veterinary health care team and the client to provide optimal care for the pet. In essence, this is a partnership, in which negotiation and shared decision making are used to take the client's perspective into consideration.[9] The key elements of effective communication include allowing the client to fully share her

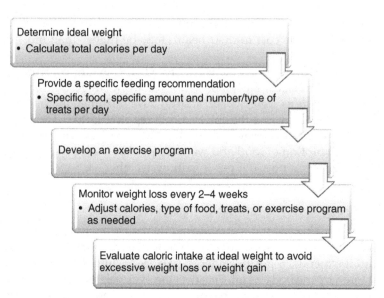

Figure 7.4. Developing a weight loss plan.

story, providing empathy and support, providing clear information, sharing decision making, and achieving agreement.[9]

Perhaps the most important component of a weight loss program is firm allegiance to the plan from everyone involved in feeding the pet. Recent work in humans has focused on the importance of teaching problem solving to help with adherence in weight loss and weight management programs.[10] In this context, problem solving can be defined as the process of developing adaptive solutions for difficult problems encountered in everyday life. Problem solving therapy (PST) focuses on teaching people specific skills to improve adaptive coping, particularly in relation to overcoming barriers to change.

As noted above, studies have shown that PST may be particularly beneficial in promoting treatment adherence. This type of therapy has been successfully applied to conditions in which therapy requires a lifestyle change such as smoking cessation and weight management programs. Adherence problems generally arise from a lack of motivation or a lack of specific skills to overcome barriers to adherence. Lack of motivation or difficulties addressing treatment obstacles often exacerbate one another. For example, in the treatment of obesity, a participant's lack of motivation to engage in regular exercise may undermine efforts to address barriers to behavioral change such as wearing a pedometer or finding a workout partner or taking the dog for a walk. PST is designed to address both the lack of motivation and the skill deficits needed to overcome barriers to adherence. While the veterinary health care team is not expected to be trained in clinical psychology,

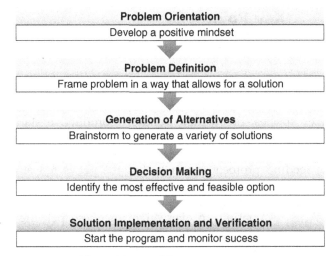

Problem Orientation

Develop a positive mindset

Problem Definition

Frame problem in a way that allows for a solution

Generation of Alternatives

Brainstorm to generate a variety of solutions

Decision Making

Identify the most effective and feasible option

Solution Implementation and Verification

Start the program and monitor sucess

Figure 7.5. Five-step problem-solving model.

they can engage pet owners with the simple five-step problem-solving model (Figure 7.5). This model is consistent with relationship centered care because it makes owners a part of the decision-making process.

For example, owners can be encouraged to develop a positive mindset by focusing on the benefits of weight loss. This may include increased quality and quantity of life for their pet or the ability to perform a specific activity or function (playing ball, jumping into the car, etc.). Calculation of current body fat percentage (Chapter 2) and determination of ideal body weight defines the problem in a concrete, nonjudgmental way that allows for a specific solution. Every client has unique circumstances; brainstorm with them to find the best weight management program. If owners are engaged in the decision-making process, they are more likely to adhere to the recommendations. After all, it was their idea too. Once the program is initiated, follow up is critical. This may include in-clinic visits, phone calls, and/or electronic communication.

Nutritional History

As discussed in Chapter 3, the veterinary health care team and the veterinary technician in particular must collect a complete nutritional history for each pet that visits their hospital. Every animal that presents to the clinic should be assessed to establish nutritional needs and feeding goals. Veterinary technicians play a key role in assessing the body condition of cats and dogs, along with the veterinarian determining if the pet needs to lose weight. Veterinary technicians also play a critical role in communicating this information to the pet owner.

Key Point

First, obtain a complete nutritional history.

The first step in evaluating an overweight pet and determining its nutritional status is to obtain a complete history, including signalment (i.e., species, breed, age, gender, reproductive status, activity level, and environment). Next, a nutritional history should be taken to determine the quality and adequacy of the food being fed to the pet, the feeding protocol (e.g., whether the pet is fed at designated meals or free choice, the amount of food given, the family member responsible for feeding the pet), and the type or types of food given. When evaluating an overweight or obese pet, the technician should ask the owner specific questions about the pet's diet. Use of a standardized diet history form facilitates collecting pertinent information.

This form includes information on the pet's access to foods, supplements, and medications, and how much of each substance the pet consumes each day. In some cases, dogs have access to commercial foods fed to cats in the household and vice versa. Pets also may be fed by more than one family member or receive numerous treats throughout the day. Determining the calorie contribution of treats to a pet's daily intake is critical. Because calorie content of common dog treats can range from 5 kcals to more than 600 kcals, some treats can contribute significantly to a dog's total daily intake. All of these factors can explain why a pet is overweight or obese. Calorie contents of typical treats are listed in Table 7.1.

Weight and body composition are determined by the nutrient composition of the pet's food and daily food intake. When reviewing the pet's nutritional history, the health care team should consider the nutrients making up the pet's diet. The caloric density of pet foods is determined by the proportion and amounts of protein, fat, and soluble carbohydrates. Caloric density is the energy/unit weight of food, usually expressed as kilocalories (kcal) or kilojoules (kJ) of metabolizable energy/gram of food, or more conveniently as calories/cup or can. The caloric density of food is crucial when selecting a diet for weight reduction. Also, the proper balance of nutrients can make the food more acceptable to the pet, which is imperative in reducing or maintaining body weight (BW).[8]

All members of the health care team should be proficient at obtaining a nutritional history. Through this mechanism, the team can pinpoint a breakdown in owner adherence (e.g., is more than one person in the household feeding the pet, is the pet getting more calories than recommended?) and begin to establish a feeding protocol to reduce the pet's calorie consumption.

Table 7.1. Calorie content of common dog treats.

Dog treats		
Manufacturer	Product	Calories/treat
Del Monte Foods	Milk Bone®	
	Original	10
	Puppy Biscuits	10
	Small Biscuits	20
	Medium Biscuits	40
	Large Biscuits	115
	Extra Large Biscuits	225
	Gravy Bones Small/Medium	35
	Gravy Bones Large	80
	Flavor Snacks Small/Medium	20
	Flavor Snacks Large	80
	Super Premium Chicken and Rice	10
	Mar-O Snacks Treat	30
	Grillin' Bites Beef Steaks	30
	Grillin' Bites Chicken Drumsticks	25
	Pup-Peroni®	24
	Snausages®	25
Purina	Beggin' Strips®	
	Bacon	30
	Cheese and Bacon	30
	Beef and Bacon	30
	Beggin' Littles (Bacon)	7
	Beggin' Wraps®	
	Bacon and Beef	18
	Bacon and Cheese	18
	Busy Bone®	
	Chew Treat Dental Small/Medium	309
	Chew Treat Dental Large	600
	Chewbone Small/ Medium	309
	Chewbone Large	618
	Chew-eez Chew Strips Savory Chicken	60
	Chew-eez Chew Strips Hearty Beef Basted	60
	Chew-eez Beefhide Rolls with Tasty Middles	
	Small	171
	Savory Chicken Large	211
	Chew-eez Chew Sticks Hearty Beef	22
	Chew-rific Twist'ems Beef and Cheese	45
	Chew-rific Twist'ems Bacon and Cheese	45
	T Bonz Sizzlin' Steak	42
	T Bonz Sizzlin' Steak and Bacon	42
	Tiny T Bonz Steak	18
	Purina One Adult Biscuits®	
	Beef and Rice	33
	Lamb and Rice	30
	Large Breed (Chicken and Rice)	84
	Healthy Weight (Turkey and Rice)	26
	Pro-Plan®	
	Adult Biscuits (Beef and Rice)	35
	Large Breed Biscuits (Chicken and Rice)	87
		(Continued)

Table 7.1. *Continued*

Mars	Pedigree®	
	BreathBuster Small	28
	BreathBuster Regular	49
	DentaBone Small	105
	DentaBone Medium	188
	DentaBone Large	300
	DentaStix Small	49
	DentaStix Regular	70
	JumBone Small	297
	JumBone Large	624
	MarroBone	39
	Puppy Trainers	5
Hill's Pet Nutrition	Science Diet®	
	Simple Essentials™ Treats	
	Immunity Support Adult Wafer Treats	27
	Immunity Support Puppy Wafer Treats	27
	Light Adult Large Biscuit with Real Chicken	58
	Light Adult Medium Biscuit with Real Chicken	31
	Mobility Adult Large Biscuit with Real Chicken	70
	Mobility Adult Medium Biscuit with Real Chicken	23
	Oral Care Adult Large Nugget	21
	Oral Care Adult Medium Nugget	10
	Skin and Coat Adult Jerky Strips with Real Beef and Vegetables	45
	Skin and Coat Adult Jerky Strips with Real Chicken and Vegetables	45
	Skin and Coat Adult Medium Biscuit with Real Chicken	23
	Skin and Coat Puppy Medium Biscuit with Real Chicken	27
	Training Adult Treats with Real Beef	9
	Prescription Diet®	
	Hypoallergenic Treats	17
	Dog Treat	14

Diagnostic Tests

One of the most difficult aspects the veterinary health care team faces is talking to clients about their pet's weight when the pet is overweight or obese. Describing a pet as overweight or obese can be similar to telling someone her child is overweight or obese. This can be a very emotional subject for both owners and the health care team. Because of the societal stigma associated with obesity in people, it can feel awkward to talk to a client about her pet's weight, particularly if the owner is also overweight. The social stigma is real, but so are the threats to health status that obesity poses. Health care team members must be empathic in their discussions regarding weight. At the same time, the health care team has a responsibility to the pet to address this disease condition.

Overweight or obese patients are suffering from a disease that is known to lead to or exacerbate other disease conditions and shorten life.

Key Point

Owners of overweight pets tend to interpret every request for attention as a request for food.

For human health care providers, calculating a body mass index (BMI) is the first step toward using a nonjudgmental, dispassionate clinical indicator to introduce the importance of weight management to a patient. Despite the fact that many human health care providers consider weight management a frustrating condition to treat, studies have shown that documenting a diagnosis of overweight or obesity has a positive effect on patients' weight loss.[11] For the veterinary health care team, it is equally important to use tools that help objectively diagnose the disease. When evaluating a purebred dog, it may be useful to review and educate the owner on the standards set for the particular breed (Table 7.2). However, there is significant variation in the ideal weight for individuals of a given breed. The most accurate and objective method of assessing body fat is to calculate the pet's ideal body weight and percent body fat as described in Chapter 2.[12,13] The ideal weight and current percent body fat provides an objective assessment of the percent of weight attributable to excess body fat. This value can be discussed with the owner in a fashion similar to any other abnormal diagnostic finding, removing the emotional aspect.

Body condition scoring (BCS) also can be a used to subjectively diagnose the pet's weight and can be used to include the client in the process. Owners can be easily taught to perform a BCS assessment on their pet so they can recognize an ideal weight for their dog based on appearance and palpation. This also takes the focus off of the owner and provides an impartial assessment of the pet's body condition. Assessing a patient's fat stores and muscle mass independent of body weight provides the health care team with a tool that can be used in team communication. The two most common BCS systems are the five-point scale and the nine-point scale. Both scales use nine points, but the five-point scale is scored to the nearest half-point, whereas the nine-point scale is scored to the whole point.[2,14] A more detailed discussion of body condition scoring can be found in Chapter 2. It is important for all members of the health care team to use the same scoring system from the outset so as not to confuse or miscalculate the patient's body condition.

Regardless of the method used to assess body fat, the health care team should document each pet's current body weight, ideal body weight, percent body fat, and/or BCS at every visit as part of the physical examination.

Table 7.2. AKC breed standard weights.

Cats

Domestic	8–10 lbs
Coon	11–15 lbs
Persian	10–11 lbs
Siamese	5–10 lbs

Weight can vary greatly within the same breed, so consider percent body fat, body condition score, age, and body size when determining if a feline patient is at a healthy weight.

Dogs
Giant breeds

Bloodhound	80–110 lbs
Borzoi	55–105 lbs
Bull Mastiff	88–130 lbs
Great Dane	121–176 lbs
Great Pyrenees	85–121 lbs
Irish Wolfhound	105–120 lbs
Mastiff	165–198 lbs
Newfoundland	110–152 lbs
Rottweiler	88–110 lbs
Saint Bernard	110–200 lbs
Scottish Deerhound	66–110 lbs

Large breeds

Afghan Hound	50–60 lbs
Alaskan Malamute	75–126 lbs
Bernese Mountain Dog	88–110 lbs
Black and Tan Coonhound	55–80 lbs
Bouvier des Flandres	60–88 lbs
Boxer	53–70 lbs
Briard	75 lbs
Chesapeake Bay Retriever	55–80 lbs
Collie	44–75 lbs
Curly-coated Retriever	70–80 lbs
Doberman Pinscher	64–88 lbs
English Foxhound	65–70 lbs
English Setter	40–70 lbs
Eskimo	55–110 lbs
Flat-coated Retriever	55–80 lbs
German Shepherd	70–95 lbs
German Shorthaired Pointer	45–70 lbs
Golden Retriever	55–75 lbs
Gordon Setter	45–80 lbs
Greyhound	60–70 lbs
Irish Setter	60–70 lbs
Irish Water Spaniel	45–65 lbs
Labrador Retriever	55–80 lbs
Old English Sheepdog	55–66 lbs
Pointer	45–75 lbs
Poodle (standard)	44–70 lbs
Rhodesian Ridgeback	70–85 lbs
Schnauzer (giant)	66–77 lbs
Weimaraner	70–85 lb

Table 7.2. *Continued*

Medium breeds

Airedale Terrier	42–55 lbs
American Water Spaniel	25–45 lbs
Basset Hound	40–60 lbs
Beagle	26–31 lbs
Border Collie	30–45 lbs
Brittany Spaniel	30–40 lbs
Bulldog	40–55 lbs
Bull Terrier	52–62 lbs
Chow Chow	44–70 lbs
Clumber Spaniel	55–85 lbs
Dalmatian	50–59 lbs
English Springer Spaniel	40–50 lbs
Field Spaniel	35–55 lbs
Harrier	48–60 lbs
Keeshond	55–66 lbs
Kerry Blue Terrier	33–40 lbs
Puli	22–33 lbs
Samoyed	37–66 lbs
Schnauzer (standard)	33–40 lbs
Siberian Husky	35–60 lbs
Staffordshire Bull Terrier	24–38 lbs
Sussex Spaniel	35–45 lbs
Welch Springer Spaniel	35–45 lbs
Wirehaired Pointing Griffon	50–60 lbs

Small breeds

Basenji	22–24 lbs
Bedlington Terrier	17–23 lbs
Border Terrier	11–16 lbs
Boston Terrier	15–25 lbs
Cairn Terrier	13–16 lbs
Dachshund (standard)	16–32 lbs
English Cocker Spaniel	26–34 lbs
Fox Terrier	15–18 lbs
French Bulldog	18–29 lbs
Irish Terrier	25–27 lbs
Lakeland Terrier	15–17 lbs
Manchester Terrier (standard)	12–16 lbs
Poodle (miniature)	11 lbs
Pug	14–18 lbs
Schipperke (small)	7–11 lbs
Schipperke (large)	11–18 lbs
Schnauzer (miniature)	11–15 lbs
Scottish Terrier	18–22 lbs
Shih Tzu	9–18 lbs
Skye Terrier	25 lbs
Smooth Fox Terrier	15–18 lbs
Welsh Corgi (Cardigan)	25–38 lbs
Welsh Corgi (Pembroke)	22–30 lbs
Welsh Terrier	20–21 lbs
West Highland White Terrier	15–22 lbs
Whippet	28 lbs

(Continued)

Table 7.2. *Continued*

Toy breeds	
Affenpinscher	6.5–9 lbs
Australian Terrier	14 lbs
Brussels Griffon	5–12 lbs
Cavalier King Charles Spaniel	10–18 lbs
Chihuahua	6 lbs
Dachshund (miniature)	11 lbs
English Toy Spaniel	8–14 lbs
Italian Greyhound	5.5–10 lbs
Maltese	4–6 lbs
Miniature Pinscher	10 lbs
Norwich Terrier	10–12 lbs
Papillon	3.3–11 lbs
Pekingese	7–14.3 lbs
Pomeranian	3–7 lbs
Silky Terrier	8–10 lbs
Yorkshire Terrier	8 lbs

These average weight ranges (in lbs) for adults of each breed are based on information from veterinary nutritionists at Hill's Pet Nutrition, Inc., and *Small Animal Clinical Nutrition*, 5th edition. These ranges should serve as a starting point for assessment. Remember, the weight of an individual animal depends on several factors such as breed, gender, body size, lifestyle, and the pet's spay or neuter status.

Determine Calorie Requirements

It is likely that the frustration many veterinary health care teams have with weight reduction programs stems from use of an inaccurate starting point. Currently most feeding plans use one of four approaches to decrease calorie intake:

- Reduction: Feed less of current food and/or eliminate snacks
- Method: Eliminate free-choice feeding
- Diet: Change to a therapeutic weight-loss or light food
- Feeding guidelines: Decrease recommendation on the bag by X%

Sadly, a recent study showed these feeding plans are wrong 75% of the time.[15] Patients, clients, and the pet are set up to fail. Basing feeding plans on an accurate ideal body weight increases success. Once the ideal body weight has been determined, the resting energy requirement (RER) and daily energy requirement (DER) can be determined.

The DER reflects the pet's activity level and is calculated based on the pet's RER for ideal weight, which is the amount of energy the pet uses at rest in a thermoneutral environment. The following formula can be used to determine the RER for a cat or dog: RER kcal/day = 70 (BW in kg)$^{0.75}$

Because adipose tissue uses very little energy for maintenance, lean body mass primarily determines DER.[1] The DER can be calculated as follows:

- Obesity-prone dog: DER = 1.4 × RER
- Overweight dog: DER = 1.0 × RER
- Obesity-prone cat: DER = 1.0 × RER
- Overweight cat: DER = 0.8 × RER

Resting energy requirements are also available from many pet food companies or in Chapter 3, Table 3.9. It is important to recommend a food appropriate for weight loss or for managing obesity-prone pets. Lesser quality foods may put the pet at risk for protein deprivation when on a weight loss program, so it is appropriate to evaluate the pet's protein needs when developing the feeding plan. A detailed discussion of therapeutic foods for weight loss can be found in Chapter 4.

Once all of the above information has been gathered, the health care team should formulate a weight loss plan that includes a specific weight loss goal, the maximum daily amount of calories allowed to meet this goal, the specific food and amount to be fed, and the way the food is to be fed (usually meal feeding vs. free choice). The plan also should include a system for monitoring the pet's weight and adjusting the caloric intake, type of food, and exercise regimen based on the observed weight loss (or lack thereof), as well as dietary guidelines to maintain the pet's weight when the ideal weight is reached. The food diary kept by the pet owner aids in evaluating weight loss and adjusting the plan as necessary.

Implementing the Program

Pet owners must pay strict attention to the foods given to their pet. Daily excesses of as little as a quarter cup (2 oz) of a calorie-restricted food can make or break a weight loss program. Treating behavior is an expression of affection from owner to pet, so it is imperative to remind pet owners that treats are part of the overall daily caloric intake and must be taken into account. Owners may not realize that many human food treats contribute significant calories to their pets' intake. For a 20-lb dog, 1 oz of cheese would be the equivalent of the owner consuming one and a half hamburgers as a treat. For a cat or smaller dog, that same amount of cheese would be the equivalent of consuming three and a half hamburgers as a treat. Providing these types of comparisons may help owners recognize the impact of and control their treating behaviors.

Figure 7.6 provides some examples of calorie content equivalents. Calorie contents of many human foods can be conveniently found at a variety of online sources including www.nutritiondata.com. Calorie contents of many commercial treats are listed in Table 7.1. In some cases

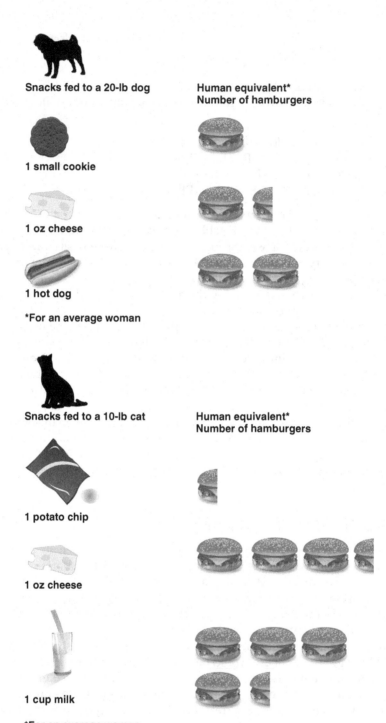

Figure 7.6. Treat translator chart. Images from Fotolia.com.

it may be necessary to contact the treat manufacturer to determine its calorie content. Encouraging owners to keep a daily food journal may help both the veterinary health care team and the owner recognize sources of excess calories.

Food Journal

Food journals have been used by many weight loss programs for people. Documenting daily food intake allows dieters to recognize and control over-consumption of calories. Studies suggest that people who write down everything they eat each day lose more weight than those who do not.[16,17] This tool also is important when developing a weight loss program for pets. The health care team should encourage the owner to keep a food journal that includes a complete account of what his pet eats each day (Figure 7.7).

In this example, Barlow is a male, neutered domestic shorthair with a current weight of 14 lbs and an ideal weight of 12 lbs. To reach his ideal

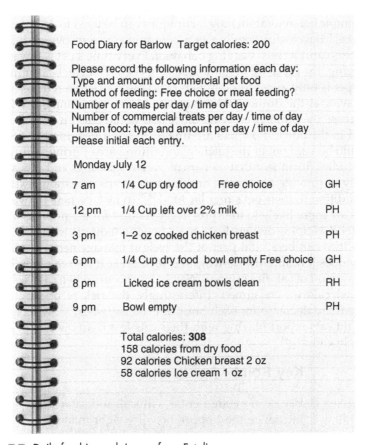

Figure 7.7. Daily food journal. Image from Fotolia.com.

weight, he must consume 80% of the RER for a 12-lb cat, which is 200 calories/day. The owners are feeding a commercial dry light food which contains 316 kcal/cup. Contributions from the human food treats were determined by consulting www.nutritiondata.com. This food journal demonstrates to the owners that those small treats add up to big calories, and although they are providing only 158 kcal from dry cat food, Barlow is consuming an additional 150 kcals worth of treats each day. No wonder he is not losing any weight.

Feeding Method

Generally speaking, owners should feed their pets at least twice/day; however, it is recommended that pets on a weight loss regimen be fed frequent small meals throughout the day. Therefore, owners whose schedules allow them to provide three or four small meals daily are encouraged to do so. The use of treat balls containing the weight loss food can provide access to multiple small meals in the owners' absence. The health care team should calculate the total amount of calories and volume of food for owners to provide in this manner.

Simple behavioral therapy techniques can be used to decrease caloric intake.[18] Successful begging is a common cause of overeating. Many owners cannot resist begging behavior. Every time a pet is rewarded for begging, the behavior is reinforced. This behavior can be diminished if the pet is only given food in its bowl. This restriction reduces begging behavior at the dinner table or couch. More importantly, it will likely decrease the number of treats, since additional effort is required to put food in the bowl. If owners are unable to resist begging behavior, pets should be kept out of the kitchen and dining area during family meals.

Studies document that owners of overweight dogs and cats are more likely to provide fresh meat and kitchen scraps or various extra treats in addition to their pet's regular food.[19,20] In fact, owners of overweight pets are more likely to interpret every request for attention as a request for food. Helping owners learn to respond to requests with play or other activities can be a vital part of the weight management program. Not only does it reduce the daily intake of calories, it also can help increase the amount of calories burned. Weight loss occurs when calories burned exceed calories consumed. Interestingly, the risk of obesity in dogs appears to decrease for each hour of exercise/week.[21] Owners of overweight cats report playing with their cats less than owners of normal-weight cats.[20]

Key Point

Use a nonjudgmental clinical indicator to introduce the importance of weight management to clients.

Exercise Programs

Physical activity is the most variable component of energy expenditure and therefore is a key aspect of weight loss programs in humans and pets.[22] Inclusion of moderate, regular physical activity in weight management programs may affect body weight in several ways, including increasing energy expenditure and contributing to an energy deficit, aiding in regulation of food intake, and increasing lean body mass. Increased physical activity also appears to result in improvements of metabolic abnormalities associated with obesity, even without significant changes in body weight. It has been shown to improve insulin sensitivity, partially reverse leptin resistance, and suppress the enhanced proinflammatory burden induced by obesity.[22] In obese humans, physical activity appears to have an effect on health-related outcomes that is separate from the effect attributable to body weight.[23] However, in people, physical activity is not the most efficient method of initial weight loss; rather, it appears to be more crucial for maintaining weight loss once it has occurred.[24]

Moderate, regular exercise is advocated in virtually all veterinary weight management programs. Despite these recommendations, the optimal amount of physical activity to prevent or manage obesity in dogs and cats has not been determined. Adding to the confusion is the fact that most dog owners already consider their dogs to be moderately to extremely active.[25]

In one survey more than half of pet owners indicated that they ensured their pet's quality of life by providing regular exercise, and 80% indicated that they provided daily exercise for their pets.[26] However, in studies designed to determine the accuracy of self-reported physical activity of people engaged in weight loss programs, patients consistently overestimated their physical activity by 50% to 300%.[27-29] It is likely that a similar discrepancy exists in the reported and actual behavior of pet owners with regard to the amount of physical activity their pets receive. This likely contributes to the difficulty in prescribing appropriate exercise for obese and overweight animals. For severely overweight animals or those with concurrent conditions such as arthritis, a supervised physical rehabilitation program may be most appropriate. Physical rehabilitation programs are discussed in detail in Chapter 6.

An exercise plan for an out-of-shape but otherwise healthy pet should begin slowly, with the activity level increasing gradually based on how much the pet can tolerate.[30] Dog owners should be encouraged to exercise with their pet, so the dog and person can exercise together and continue to strengthen the human-animal bond while getting fit. Walking is a simple way to burn calories and tone muscles. It also is a good way to get fit without excessive impact on joints or muscles.[31] For the owner, walking at a moderate to vigorous pace for 30 minutes burns 140 to 230 calories in a 154-lb person.

The benefits of people and pets exercising together have been studied. Results document that when owners participate in a weight loss program with their dog, they are more likely to continue participating in the program.[32] In this study participants also reported that exercising with their pets resulted in a significantly greater enhancement of their own quality of life. A separate study documented that dog walking promotes physical activity and contributes to weight control in people. This study found that dog walkers were more likely to meet the national recommendations for moderate to vigorous physical activity compared to people who had but did not walk their dogs and those who did not own dogs.[33] Indeed, there were significantly fewer obese dog walkers (17%) when compared to both owners who did not walk their dogs (28%) and non-owners (22%).[33]

A dog's playful, carefree nature is contagious. Who can resist his dog when it brings a toy, ball, or frisbee? Owners should heed this advice and take time to play to alleviate stresses from home, work, and everyday life. The amazing thing about playing with a dog is that it is exercise in a fun atmosphere, and it can occur just about anytime or anywhere.

Veterinary technicians must communicate this to owners and encourage them to engage in a variety of play activities with their pets. Throwing a ball for their dog to chase is a great activity for owners with any size yard. Playing fetch helps the dog with its natural instinct to chase and retrieve prey. Dogs and humans love adventure, so consider recommending that clients take a hike with their dogs. Hiking can burn close to 400 calories/hour for the average person.

Exercising with dogs can be fun for the whole family. Children can and should get involved with the four-legged "kids" in the family. Children can interact with pets in activities similar to those already mentioned. Families can also get involved in agility, flyball, frisbee, and breed-specific activities such as herding. Many local 4-H programs involve the family, and the family pets can be the main component of a 4-H program or project. Interestingly, a recent study documented that both boys and girls in dog-owning homes consistently had a higher level of physical activity than those from homes without a dog.[34] The researchers suggest that children with dogs were accompanying their parents when walking the dog or playing with the dog at home rather than playing on the computer or watching television. This increased activity could mean a significant difference for both the dog's and the children's long term health. As with any exercise program, it is important to remind owners that the endurance of both the dog and the owner must be built gradually.

Cat owners must be more creative when trying to increase their pets' activity level. One study has demonstrated that environmental enrichment increased activity and weight loss in overweight cats in a multi-cat household.[35] Owners can enrich their cats' environments by adding climbing towers and scratching posts to encourage natural feline behaviors. Toys (e.g., laser pointers, feather toys, noisy balls) and grooming tools can help to increase a cat's overall wellness and the time they spend with their owners. In this study, owners who participated in the environmental enrichment group had a more positive image of their cat and felt they were playing a more active role in their cat's health. Overall, these results suggest that increasing activity while restricting food intake may improve the outcome of obesity therapy of cats and simultaneously enhance client satisfaction with the interventions. Environmental enrichment is a practical and simple method to help cats lose weight that can be tailored to the individual's lifestyle and resources.

Activity also can be increased by taking advantage of cats' natural instinct to hunt prey. Instead of providing all of their cat's food in one location, owners can make their cat hunt for it. During the day, provide one-half of the total caloric intake for the day divided into small portions, then place these in various locations throughout the house—on bookshelves, on different floors of the house, and in hidden areas—to entice the cats to hunt for their food. Figure 7.8 provides an estimate of calories burned for a variety of activities in dogs and cats.

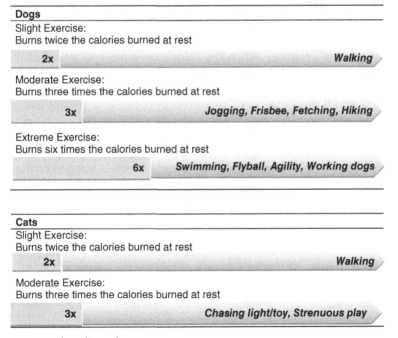

Figure 7.8. Calorie burn chart.

Monitoring and Adjusting the Program

Re-check visits to monitor the patient's weight loss are important to ensure the program is working and to motivate the pet owner to continue. To ensure success, the pet must be assessed at three critical points: the beginning of the program, the end of the program, and during a plateau in weight loss. The pet owner must be encouraged and complimented when her pet loses weight. Encouraging the owner is important, even when the pet's weight remains constant or increases from visit to visit. When the pet fails to make progress, many owners may become discouraged and decide to abandon the therapy. When a pet fails to lose weight while on a weight loss program, the reason must be determined and explained to the pet owner. Possible reasons for lack of progress and potential solutions are outlined in Figure 7.9.

Regular monitoring and counseling at re-check visits are the most efficient ways of avoiding problems with weight loss. The best reinforcement for owner compliance is a visible reduction in their pet's body weight and a subsequent return of normal body contours, and resolution of clinical signs that may be present. Charting the pet's progress toward its ideal body weight can provide encouragement to the owners (Figure 7.10). Weight loss in dogs and cats is most readily seen as a decrease in pelvic or abdominal circumference. Successful weight loss can be tracked by measuring pelvic and thoracic circumference at each re-check and periodically reassessing BCS.

Re-checks should be scheduled to allow enough time for visible progress. Shorter intervals are needed at the beginning and end of a weight loss program, when the caloric contents and amounts of food may require more frequent adjusting. The first re-check usually can be scheduled for two weeks after the initiation of the program. Cats and some small dogs may need three weeks before any weight loss can be measured. No more than four weeks should pass before the pet is re-checked. A reasonable estimate of weight loss in dogs and cats is 2% loss of initial body weight/week.[1] From the owner's perspective, a rate of at least 0.5% of the initial body weight/week is needed to maintain owner interest in completing the weight loss program. Pets that are truly obese and have slower metabolic rates may need to maintain the

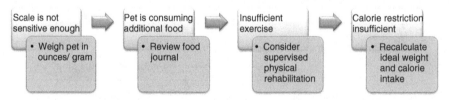

Figure 7.9. Common causes for lack of weight loss.

Client:	Judy Thompson	Date of Assessment: 06-07-2010
Patient:	**Gracie**	
Age:	7 years	Date of Follow-Up: _____
Breed:	Labrador Retriever	
Current Weight:	105.0 lbs.	
Current Index	56%	

At 105 pounds, Gracie has a **high risk** for serious weight-related health conditions such as:
- Diabetes
- Heart disease
- Arthritis
- Physical injuries
- Shortened life expectancy

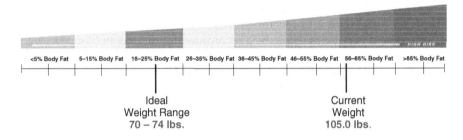

| <5% Body Fat | 5–15% Body Fat | 16–25% Body Fat | 26–35% Body Fat | 36–45% Body Fat | 46–55% Body Fat | 56–65% Body Fat | >65% Body Fat |

Ideal
Weight Range
70 – 74 lbs.

Current
Weight
105.0 lbs.

Now more than ever it's important to get your pet to a healthy weight. Please talk to your veterinarian today about a program to get Gracie to a healthy weight and reduce her risks for weight related diseases.

Figure 7.10. Chart pet's progress toward ideal weight.

weight loss program for eight to 12 months. The staff must educate owners on this timeline to ensure compliance and success.

Following Up

Approximately 55% of overweight dogs and cats are not brought back for a weight loss follow-up visit, which is a disturbing statistic considering that pets returning for three or more visits have been found to be successful in losing weight.[14,30] Re-check visits provide another opportunity for the health care team to stress to the owner how important the program is in maintaining or restoring the pet's health. These follow-up visits also reinforce the client's commitment to the pet's weight loss program by allowing the owner to see the results of his or her efforts; without this positive reinforcement, the owner may not continue with the program. In humans, people who attend support groups or regular recheck visit as part of their weight loss programs lose more weight and maintain weight loss longer than those who did not.[36,37] Finally, re-check visits allow the staff to adjust the caloric intake, feeding plan, and exercise regimen if needed for the program's continued success. Multiple modes of reminders—phone, mail, or electronic—should be used to increase adherence to re-check appointments.

Communication has been the theme for veterinary technicians thus far throughout this chapter. Communication seems to be the technician's task that makes or breaks compliance on the part of the owner. To optimize the success of a weight management program, the $C = R + A + FT$ formula (Compliance = Recommendation + Acceptance + Follow-Through) is imperative.[38] Compliance is the measure of whether the pets seen in the hospital actually receive the care that the health care team and the profession believe is best for them. Is the recommendation that was made for the patient by the veterinarian being followed by the owner?

Recommendation involves taking all of the diagnostic information (ideal body weight, current body weight, BCS, history, physical exam, etc.) into account and recommending a solution. However, often what the health care team thinks is a recommendation may not be perceived as such by the owner. Simply stating "switch Fido to a light food and follow the directions on the bag and let us know if you have any problems or questions" is NOT a recommendation. There are too many potential problems with this statement. Recommendations must be as specific as possible—which food, how much to feed, when to feed, how to feed, etc.—and should be in writing. Veterinary technicians should then follow up with the client by calling to see how the transition is going, if there any questions, etc.

The next part of the formula involves acceptance. This is probably the most crucial part of the $C = R + A + FT$ formula. The veterinary technician discusses obesity and the health risks associated with obesity with the client. The recommendation made by the veterinarian is reinforced by the technician. This recommendation is again reviewed. The dialogue between technician and owner is critical to a successful weight management program. This discussion is aimed at ensuring the client understands the recommendation, why it was made, the impact of the disease condition on the pet, and the treatment plan. If any of these are missed or misunderstood, the owner likely will not be compliant with the recommendation.

The final piece to compliance is follow-through. Follow-through involves re-checks (having the patient return to the hospital for weight assessments). The first re-check appointment should be made before the client even leaves the hospital. Re-check appointments were discussed earlier in this chapter, but it should be reiterated that the veterinary technician should call the client in three to five days to discuss the feeding transition, treating, the exercise regimen, and any other questions that may have arisen since the hospital visit and recommendation. Another helpful tool is to send a repurchase reminder to the client to let him know that he will run low on food (due to the calculations you sent home) and it is time to purchase another bag. It is important to remember that roughly 55% of overweight dogs and cats are not brought back for a weight loss follow-up visit. Again, it is a disturbing statistic, considering that pets returning for three or more visits have been found to be successful in losing weight.[14,30]

Summary

Companion animals have truly become just that—our companions. They love their humans unconditionally and in return they receive love, health care, nutrition, and most importantly, the achievement of family member status. Having become true members of the family also leads to sharing the lifestyle of the family, its eating habits. The epidemic of obesity in America has been shared with our pets, and the ever increasing percentage of overweight or obese companion animals is alarming. However, the veterinary health care team can and should be responsible for helping to halt this growing disease condition. Identifying and diagnosing this condition, setting up a treatment plan, gaining the owner's understanding and acceptance, and following up with the patient and owner will start that pet and the rest of the population on the road to weight management. Pet owners love their pets. It is the health care team's responsibility to make sure they do not love them to death and put the patient (and often the owner) on the path to better health.

References

1. Toll PW, Yamka RM, Schoenherr WD, et al. 2010. Obesity. In: Hand MS, Thatcher CD, Remillard RL, et al., eds. *Small Animal Clinical Nutrition*, 5th ed. Topeka, KS: Mark Morris Institute, 501–535.
2. Armstrong PJ, Lund EM. 1996. Changes in body composition and energy balance with aging. *Veterinary Clinical Nutrition* 3:83–87.
3. Burkholder WJ, Toll PW. 2000. Obesity. In: Hand MS, Thatcher CD, Remillard RL, et al., eds. *Small Animal Clinical Nutrition*, 4th ed. Topeka, KS: Mark Morris Institute, 401–430.
4. German AJ. 2010. Obesity, Biology and Management. In: Ettinger SJ, Feldman EC, eds. *Textbook of Veterinary Internal Medicine*. St. Louis, MO: Saunders Elsevier, 121–124.
5. Buffington CAT. 2000. Obesity and Cachexi.a In: Fenner WR, ed. *Quick Reference to Veterinary Medicine*. Philadelphia, PA: Lippincott, Williams and Wilkins, 100–105.
6. Becker M, Kushner R. 2006. The People and Pets Health Connection. *Fitness Unleashed! A Dog Owner's Guide to Losing Weight and Gaining Health Together.* New York, NY: Three Rivers Press, 15–17.
7. Habits and Practices of Pet Owners: Hill's Pet Nutrition, Inc., 2002.
8. Flegal KM, Carroll MD, Ogden CL, et al. 2002. Prevalence and trends in obesity among US adults, 1999–2000. *JAMA* 288:1723–1727.

9. Shaw JR, Adams CL, Bonnett BN. 2004. What can veterinarians learn from studies of physician-patient communication about veterinarian-client-patient communication? *J Am Vet Med Assoc* 224:676–684.

10. Murawski ME, Milsom VA, Ross KM, et al. 2009. Problem solving, treatment adherence, and weight-loss outcome among women participating in lifestyle treatment for obesity. *Eat Behav* 10:146–151.

11. Lemay CA, Cashman S, Savageau J, et al. 2003. Underdiagnosis of obesity at a community health center. *J Am Board Fam Pract* 16:14–21.

12. Lusby AL, Kirk CA, Toll PW, et al. 2010. Effectiveness of BCS for estimation of ideal body weight and energy requirements in overweight and obese dogs compared to DXA (abstract). *Journal of Veterinary Internal Medicine* 24:717.

13. Toll PW, Paetau-Robinson I, Lusby AL, et al. 2010. Effectiveness of morphometric measurements for predicting body composition in overweight and obese dogs. *Journal of Veterinary Internal Medicine* 24:717.

14. Remillard RL. 2005. Obesity. In: Ettinger SJ, Feldman EC, eds. *Textbook of Veterinary Internal Medicine, Diseases of the Dog and Cat*. Philadelphia: WB Saunders, 76–78.

15. Linder DE, Freeman LM. 2010. Evaluation of calorie density and feeding directions for commercially available diets designed for weight loss in dogs and cats. *J Am Vet Med Assoc* 236:74–77.

16. Burke LE, Sereika SM, Music E, et al. 2008. Using instrumented paper diaries to document self-monitoring patterns in weight loss. *Contemp Clin Trials* 29:182–193.

17. Wadden TA, Berkowitz RI, Womble LG, et al. 2005. Randomized trial of lifestyle modification and pharmacotherapy for obesity. *N Engl J Med* 353:2111–2120.

18. Norris MP, Beaver BV. 1993. Application of behavior therapy techniques to the treatment of obesity in companion animals. *J Am Vet Med Assoc* 202:728–730.

19. Kienzle E, Bergler R, Mandernach A. 1998. A comparison of the feeding behavior and the human-animal relationship in owners of normal and obese dogs. *J Nutr* 128:2779S–2782S.

20. Kienzle E, Bergler R. 2006. Human-animal relationship of owners of normal and overweight cats. *Journal of Nutrition* 136:1947S–1950S.

21. Robertson ID. 2003. The association of exercise, diet and other factors with owner-perceived obesity in privately owned dogs from metropolitan Perth, WA. *Prev Vet Med* 58:75–83.

22. Roudebush P, Schoenherr WD, Delaney SJ. 2008. An evidence-based review of the use of therapeutic foods, owner education, exercise, and drugs for the management of obese and overweight pets. *J Am Vet Med Assoc* 233:717–725.

23. Jakicic J, Otto A. 2005. Physical activity considerations for the treatment and prevention of obesity. *Am J Clin Nutr* 82:226S–229S.

24. Scheen AJ. 2002. Results of obesity treatment. *Ann Endocrinol (Paris)* 63:163–170.

25. Slater MR, Robinson LE, Zoran DL, et al. 1995. Diet and exercise patterns in pet dogs. *J Am Vet Med Assoc* 207:186–190.
26. American Animal Hospital Association. AAHA 2004 *pet owner survey.* www.aahanet.org. Accessed July 9, 2010.
27. Forbes GB. 1993. Diet and exercise in obese subjects: Self-report versus controlled measurements. *Nutr Rev* 51:296–300.
28. Lichtman SW, Pisarska K, Berman ER, et al. 1992. Discrepancy between self-reported and actual caloric intake and exercise in obese subjects. *N Engl J Med* 327:1893–1898.
29. Klesges RC, Eck LH, Mellon MW, et al. 1990. The accuracy of self-reports of physical activity. *Med Sci Sports Exerc* 22:690–697.
30. Burns KM. 2006. Managing overweight or obese pets. *Veterinary Technician* June:385–389.
31. Moore A. 2004. *Healthy Dog: The Ultimate Fitness Guide for You and Your Dog.* Irvine, CA: Bowtie Press.
32. Kushner RF, Blatner DJ, Jewell DE, et al. 2006. The PPET Study: People and pets exercising together. *Obesity (Silver Spring)* 14:1762–1770.
33. Coleman KJ, Rosenberg DE, Conway TL, et al. 2008. Physical activity, weight status, and neighborhood characteristics of dog walkers. *Prev Med* 47:309–312.
34. Owen CG, Nightingale CM, Rudnicka AR, et al. 2010. Family dog ownership and levels of physical activity in childhood: Findings from the Child Heart and Health Study in England. *Am J Public Health* 100:1669–1671.
35. Trippany JR, Funk J, Buffinton CA. 2003. Effects of environmental enrichments on weight loss in cats. *J Vet Intern Med* 17:430.
36. Orth WS, Madan AK, Taddeucci RJ, et al. 2008. Support group meeting attendance is associated with better weight loss. *Obes Surg* 18:391–394.
37. ter Bogt NC, Bemelmans WJ, Beltman FW, et al. 2009. Preventing weight gain: One-year results of a randomized lifestyle intervention. *Am J Prev Med* 37:270–277.
38. AAHA. 2003. The Compliance Equation. In: Grieve GA, Neuhoff KT, Thomas RM, et al., eds. *The Path to High-Quality Care: Practical Tips for Improving Compliance.* Denver, CO: American Animal Hospital Association.

Implementing a Weight Management Program

Rebecca L. Remillard, PhD, DVM, DACVN

How often have you heard clients complain, "That weight loss food you recommended just doesn't work" or "I've tried to get my dog/cat to lose weight but nothing seems to help"? How often is it true that those same clients never came back for a scheduled recheck or to pick up the next bag of therapeutic weight loss food? One of the most frustrating aspects of weight management programs is convincing owners to follow recommendations made by the health care team. "Since AAHA conducted the profession's first landmark study on compliance in 2002, the veterinary profession has seen a groundswell of awareness in terms of compliance, particularly as a driver of quality care and economic benefit. Practices now accept greater responsibility for compliance and understand that the actions of practice team members can significantly affect pet owner behaviors."[1]

Getting Started

As with any journey, quest, or goal, it is important at the beginning to believe in the worthiness of the end result. Veterinarians, as a group, have difficulty discussing obesity with pet owners because of the possible personal ramifications for both the client and health care team. Veterinarians have little to no problem explaining heartworm disease to an owner, most likely because it is a relatively detached nonemotional issue. A veterinarian may be more passionate when explaining Lyme disease to a pet owner if she has actually experienced the symptoms. However, explaining the short- and long-term consequences of obesity to pet owners does not come easily for most health care members.

Practical Weight Management in Dogs and Cats, First Edition. Edited by Todd L. Towell.
© 2011 John Wiley and Sons, Inc. Published 2011 by John Wiley & Sons, Inc.

This iatrogenic disease is present in at least 34% of the U.S. population (ages 20 to 74 yrs).[2] Discussing pet obesity can be difficult when facing an overweight client or when the veterinarian and/or staff members are overweight. Hence, getting started on any pet weight loss program for the practice begins at home. The health care team must first "heal thyself."

Staff Training

Veterinarians and health care teams in general lack knowledge and conviction regarding weight management, and are therefore relatively ineffective when attempting to impress upon owners the importance of achieving optimal body weight. With knowledge comes conviction; therefore, it is important to begin the practice weight management program in the hospital.

> ### Key Point
>
> Start the weight management program in the hospital first.

Begin with a short series of "lunch and learns" during which reader-friendly articles that present the biomechanical and metabolic changes associated with obesity in both humans and animals are reviewed. Most members of the health care team are poorly educated about their own diet and nutrition. Having a local dietitian or Weight Watchers® coach in for lunch may raise the team's level of interest and awareness. Weight management is not just about calories in, but about calories out as well. Therefore, developing group activities such as biking, hiking, or participating in a local "fun run" or a regular weekly session at the gym raises the issue of exercise to a level of importance. Having a physically fit and educated health care team accomplishes several things:

1. The personal benefits gained from weight loss and increased activity motivate the team through first-hand experience.
2. The objective information collectively gained empowers the team to have conviction about the benefits of weight loss to the pet. For example, members of the health care team may learn that adipose tissue is a complex endocrine organ that releases a variety of adipokines that regulate energy metabolism, cardiovascular function, reproductive status, and immune function.[3] Abnormal production of adipokines in obese subjects has been linked to co-morbidities such as diabetes, metabolic syndrome, cancer, and probably pancreatitis.
3. Because there are many similarities between pet and human obesity, the information directed toward the pet also applies to the owner;

therefore, discussing obese pets should be educational for the owner on several levels.

Conduct an in-hospital trial run of the program before implementing a pet owner weight loss program. Conduct a "biggest loser or winner" contest using employee pets to test the program's logistics.

Implementing the Program

The ideal weight loss program includes three components: diet, exercise, and support.

> ### Key Point
>
> Components of an ideal program include diet, exercise, and support.

Diet

The ideal weight loss diet is restricted in calories while meeting the pet's non-energy nutrient requirements. Ideally, only body fat should be lost, while lean tissue and bone are preserved. Based on several weight loss studies performed in both dogs and cats, it appears that a high-protein, high-fiber (mixture of soluble and insoluble) diet specifically supplemented with carnitine is efficacious for most overweight or obese pets.[4,5]

A therapeutic weight loss diet should be prescribed with a daily food dosage written out for the owner to take home. Calculating the food dosage is much easier when using one of several free, easy-to-use software programs available from companies that sell therapeutic weight loss diets (Hill's Pet Nutrition, Purina, Royal Canin).

For overweight cats and dogs less than 25 lbs, dry weight loss diets should be measured in specific 1/4- or 1/3-cup portions, and canned foods must be measured in teaspoons. For overweight dogs less than 5 lbs, counting kibbles for each meal is recommended and is reasonably successful. Better yet, for all body weights, using a gram food scale increases accuracy and success. The food offered at each meal should be weighed on a gram scale, especially if the meal size is less than 1 cup or 1 can of food. There can be as much as 20% variability in the amount measured by different people, which could be the difference between weight loss success and failure.[5]

> ### Key Point
>
> Measuring cups result in 20% variability from day to day.

Food scales that weigh in grams can be purchased from local grocery stores, large discount retailers, wholesale clubs, or online. They range in price from $10 to $30.

A timed feeder that doles out a specific amount of dry food (in 1/4 cup measurements) at three designated times/day is very useful. The owner can then focus on maintaining the feeder and monitoring the number of meals fed while the feeder consistently delivers portion-controlled meals. Le Bistro is a timed portion-control feeder that dispenses as little as 1/4 cup/meal (www.petmate.com).

Some owners also have had success with prepackaged meals. In this case, all of the individual meals needed for one week are packaged by weight at one point in time, perhaps by someone unemotionally attached to the pet.

Treats are a fact of life, so healthy treat alternatives are a necessary component for most owners. Having owners keep a food diary is particularly helpful in this regard. A diary can be used to check daily calorie intake (food given or stolen). An owner may be less inclined to offer additional food or treats beyond the agreed upon amount if he is compelled to record that food intake. In people, use of food diaries is associated with a decrease in food intake and subsequent weight loss.[6] A daily food diary also aids in documenting food refusal by a dog when determining the effective dose of an appetite suppressant medication.

In addition to prescribing a specific diet and food dosage, estimating body fat percent (body condition score or percent body fat) and determining the rate of weight loss and optimal body weight target for a patient can be challenging. With training and practice, the health care team becomes more consistent and homogenous in their recommendations. Body condition score charts are readily available and online from pet food companies.

Often, the owner will ask for the target optimal body weight at the start of the weight loss program. Because optimal weight is difficult to estimate, it may be more reasonable to talk about body condition score (ideal percent body fat). In general, there is a loss of about 20% in body weight and a loss of about 10% in body fat for each decrease in body condition score (Table 8.1).[7]

Table 8.1. Body condition score.

BCS	Description	% Body fat
1	Thin	Less than 10
2	Underweight	10–20
3	Optimal	20
4	Overweight	20–30
5	Obese	More than 30

Remember, one of the limitations of BCS is that it is possible for a morbidly obese pet to have more than 40% body fat (i.e., a 22-lb domestic shorthair cat with an estimated optimal body weight of 12 lbs would have approximately 10 lbs of fat, which is equal to 45% body fat). In morbidly obese patients, it may be useful to use an expanded BCS system, as described in Chapter 2.

It also should be understood that although clinical weight loss programs have been shown to be successful, many have rates of weight loss slower than those published from research colonies. This discrepancy arises because client-owned pets may be heavier than research animals at the start, and unlike the research setting, noncompliance may be an issue in client households.[5,8] The expected rate of weight loss for overweight or obese client-owned dogs and cats is between 0.5% and 1% of current body weight/week.

Exercise

A regular exercise regime helps preserve lean muscle mass in the face of total weight loss. Increasing lean muscle mass also increases the daily caloric requirement, further aiding body fat loss. The benefits of a regular exercise program for dogs also extend to the owners. Studies document that dog ownership is associated with increased activity and that companion dogs can serve as social support during weight loss in people.[9,10] A walking/running/biking program implemented for both the owner and dog that is designed in consultation with a veterinarian and medical doctor, clinical physiologist, or licensed trainer from a local fitness club is ideal. In exchange, fitness clubs promoting weight loss programs for people without dogs may consider working with local shelters and humane societies to provide exercise for the overweight dogs that rarely are walked enough. For more information about a walking/running/biking program for owner and dog and canine exercise tips and suggestions from Dr. Susan Nelson, see *Science Daily*, September 10, 2009, www.sciencedaily.com.

The frequency and quality of exercise between households with a dog that is normal weight (daily) vs. overweight or obese (weekly) was found to be significant.[11] Owners who indicated that their dog was confined to a yard as its exercise rather than walked also were more likely to have an overweight or obese dog. Whenever possible, give an exercise prescription; for example, walk one mile in 20 minutes twice daily, and then either increase the distance or shorten the time at each subsequent visit if the dog was able to perform the exercise without deleterious effects.

Support

Support should be provided through a dedicated staff member, professional counseling, and social opportunities.

Nutrition Technician Concept

A trained health care team providing the same message is critical because it provides consistent and accurate information to the client. In addition, having one or two individuals dedicated to the weight loss program is most efficient, similar in concept to having a dental or radiology technician. This staff member monitors individual pets' progress and speaks with owners directly about re-check visits, rescheduling missed appointments, questions during the food transition period, ordering and picking up food refills, and the chief complaint of "acting hungry." Dietary energy restriction is necessary for weight loss, and owners often complain about hunger behavior, stealing food, and/or dissatisfaction with the small volume of food offered. This in turn puts a strain on the owner-animal bond and most often results in noncompliance or complete withdrawal from the program. Frequent contact with the owner to explain, reassure, and offer suggestions is consistent with a successful weight loss program.

Regular Check-ins

Monthly veterinary re-check visits with a two-week follow-up phone call early in the program and whenever the client is having trouble sticking to the program help many clients. For inspiration and support, invite all clients with pets on a weight loss program to meet weekly as a group, similar to dog training classes. The following suggestions may be incorporated into weekly meetings:

- Include time for success stories, exchange of successful tips, and organized group walks.
- If the practice provides a gram food scale, prepare weekly dry food meals in advance, when motivation and supervision are readily available.
- Offer a short lecture series to provide an opportunity for the health care team to share information on pet nutrition, exercise, and obesity-related disease prevention.
- Arrange short presentations on human diet and nutrition with graduate students at schools of nutrition, local coaches involved in national weight loss programs, or dietitians from local hospitals.

Cat Specifics

It is no secret it is more difficult to get cats to lose weight than it is for dogs. However, there are a few additional tips which may work for cats requiring a weight loss program:

1. Obese indoor cats almost certainly consume 250 or more kcal/day. A simple initial calculation for a feline weight loss program is to recommend feeding only 200 kcal daily for one month. On average, cats lose 1/4 to 1/2 pound/month. Therefore, weigh-ins should be scheduled monthly, using a gram scale or one with at least 1/8-lb increments. If the weight plateaus for two months, reduce the calorie intake to 175 kcal/day at the first plateau, then 150 kcal/day at the following recheck if there has been no weight loss.[12,13]

2. Cats fed therapeutic weight loss diets must be monitored carefully to ensure they are eating the allotment of food. If diet changes are made too quickly, a cat may refuse to eat the new diet, which puts it at risk for hepatic lipidosis. However, it is very rare that a cat that eats the allotted amount of a weight loss food will develop hepatic lipidosis. If the cat eats some food every day and has no other underlying disease, it is very unlikely that it will develop hepatic lipidosis while on a 150- to 200-kcal/day weight loss program.

3. Multiple-cat households are particularly challenging. When individual cat meal feeding is not possible, a generally workable recommendation is to feed the lowest calorically dense dry cat food using a limited amount, offered by free access (i.e., a certain amount of feed appropriate for the total number of cats in the house is offered free choice every 12 or 24 hours). All cats are weighed and monitored for one to two months, and underweight cats may then be offered a high-calorie canned food as a meal, temporarily separated from the group each day, to maintain an optimal body weight.

Weight Maintenance Program Examples

There are many different ways in which a practice may implement a weight maintenance program. The following examples, in total or in part, may work in certain practices. Please note that each practice must tailor the program to its staff and clients.

*   Fitness Unleashed, by Marty Becker, DVM, and Robert Kushner, MD, outlines a program for both dogs and people who need to lose weight.[14] The program was developed from the Northwestern University and Hill's Pet Nutrition People and Pets Exercising Together (PPET) study. The PPET study is the first program to demonstrate the effectiveness of a combined people and dog weight loss program. This fresh approach to the dual obesity epidemic builds on the human-companion animal bond.[10]

*   Oradell Animal Hospital begins with a 30-minute nutrition consult in which the owner completes a two-page diet history form (available at Oradell.com, under Services and Nutritional Counseling). The medical history is reviewed, a physical examination is

performed, and the pet's body weight and condition are determined by a veterinarian. A specific diet recommendation including amounts of food to feed/day is made. Owners who agree to enroll their pet in the weight loss program pay one fee, which includes five monthly 15-minute re-check appointments for weigh-ins and food dosage adjustments. The hospital lends a scale for 24 hours to cat owners who do not want to bring their cats to the hospital for the re-check visits. The follow-up for cats is then completed by phone.

- Angell Animal Medical Center has completed several weight loss studies and conducts a regular weight loss program. In general, the program includes an initial 30-minute visit to determine the source of all calorie intake, estimate the average total daily intake, and compare that to the actual daily calories required for weight loss. The conversation then focuses on the owner determining and then agreeing to how calories will be restricted. A written diet plan is designed, describing a daily food dosage with specifically allowed treats. A two-week follow-up phone call and the first monthly re-check visit dates are set before the client leaves the exam room. Reminder phone calls are made 24 to 48 hours before appointments.

- A feline weight loss study has demonstrated that conventional weight management therapy is possible in naturally occurring obese client-owned cats.[12] The weight loss program using both canned and dry food is well described with monitoring, follow-up visits, dedicated staff members, and outcomes. Key lifestyle altera-tion recommendations include education for the owner on prevent-ing excessive food intake (including limiting treats), strategies for providing non-food-related rewards, and increasing activity in the home (e.g., moving food bowls prior to meal times and organized play sessions). Exact recommendations for each pet were custom-ized based on cat (signalment, concurrent diseases) and owner (life-style, personal circumstances) factors.

Keys to Success

A key step to getting patients started on a weight loss program is con-vincing the owner that the pet is harmed by the excessive weight. This is possibly the greatest challenge. In a survey of owners of overweight pets, 52% did not agree that their pet was overweight or obese, as explained to them by a veterinary nutritionist; if the owners agreed that the pet was overweight, they did not believe that the excessive weight was harmful.[15]

Similarly, two surveys commissioned by Pfizer Animal Health in 2006 showed a significant discrepancy between perception and reality. Only 17% of dog owners considered their dogs to be overweight or obese, whereas veterinarians estimated that 47% of their client's pets had weight issues. Studies in France and New Zealand found a similar disconnect between cat owners' and veterinarians' assessments of the cat's health risks associated with the excess weight, and owner's under-estimation of the cats' percent body fat.[16,17] Interestingly, one study also found that the evaluation of overweight cats' body condition by their owners was better with a visual scale than with a verbal description.

The use of pictures is a common aspect of several successful programs. These may include:

- Body condition score charts
- Abdominal radiographs of a 20-lb cat to visualize the intra-abdominal fat
- Before and after weight loss pictures of pets of similar weight
- Videos of pets before and after weight loss, illustrating increased mobility and human interactions
- Graphic illustration of the results of the 15-year Canine Longevity Study in which Labradors maintained at healthy weight lived an average of two years (13%) longer than their overweight littermates[18]

The single most effective weight loss tool in a weight loss program appears to be re-check visits.[19] In one study, over a three-year period, 81 patients were seen and started on a weight loss program; 54% of feline patients were not returned for a re-check visit, and 56% of canine patients were not returned for a re-check visit. Those patients that were returned for three or more re-check visits lost weight.[8] Re-check appointments every two to four weeks are essential for addressing problems that arise in the household, adjusting the food dosage, and conducting weigh-ins on the same scale to monitor progress. Decreasing the daily food dosage is a necessary component to a successful weight loss program in the majority of cases.

Re-check visits with the veterinarian are important for owner reaffirmation, whereas phone call check-ups and reminders are best handled by a dedicated support staff member. Be sure to inform the owner up front that for weight loss to continue, regular re-checks to recalculate and adjust the food dosage are essential and that it will take six to 12 months to achieve optimal body weight.

Key Point

Re-check appointments are critical to success-ful weight loss programs.

Other Tips for Success

Always check for hormonal diseases (make no assumptions; check thyroid, serum liver enzymes and electrolytes, urine glucose) before instituting a weight loss program. Often, a weight loss program is still needed once the hormonal abnormalities have been corrected, but weight loss always should follow treatment for the hormone disorder, not vice versa.

If a pet must lose more than 5% of its body weight to achieve optimal body weight, recommend a therapeutic diet to ensure nutritional balance. No over-the-counter "weight control," "weight management," or "light" diet is properly balanced nutritionally to strategically meet the pet's non-energy nutrient requirements while producing a caloric deficiency.

In one study, the mean number of people in the household caring for the pet was significantly higher for overweight or obese dogs than normal weight dogs.[11] Hence, there is now evidence to complement the clinical impression that weight loss programs are more successful if one member of the household takes total responsibility for feeding the pet.

In dogs, if aggressive behaviors related to hunger prevent successful weight loss, institute appetite suppression (Slentrol®, Pfizer Animal Health). This gives the owner time to implement the feeding program and return the dog's weight to ideal before having to manage appetite-related behaviors. Appetite suppression was possible in the majority (more than 75%) of dogs in a weight loss study conducted at Angell Animal Medical Center (author observations, study in progress).

Achieving an ideal body condition score is not always necessary or possible to achieve a health benefit. There are many benefits to losing weight when stabilized at a BCS of 3.5/5. In the life span study, dogs with BCS 6/9 lived longer than the littermates at BCS 7/9.[18] Most cats appear to avoid the orthopedic and metabolic co-morbidities by reaching 18 lbs or less (author observation).

Online Tools

PetFit.com is an alliance between the American Veterinary Medical Association (AVMA) and Hill's Pet Nutrition dedicated to using education to fight the growing pet obesity epidemic. The AVMA and Hill's focus on raising awareness about the correct way to achieve and maintain healthy weight through proper diet, exercise, and regular veterinary guidance.

www.vet.ohio-state.edu/indoorcat.htm was created to enrich the lives of indoor cats. Given that indoor enrichment is as important as an excellent diet and health care, this website discusses what it means to be a cat, advises owners about the unique needs of indoor cats, troubleshoots problems, and has ideas for increasing the activity of indoor cats.

www.stopcanineobesity.com offers a body assessment rating for canines (BARC) survey with nine questions to help dog owners determine their dog's risk for obesity, and directs them to discuss these specific points with their veterinarian.

www.petobesityprevention.com, the website of the Association for Pet Obesity Prevention (APOP), offers a variety of tools and articles in an owner-friendly format. The site offers an online pet weight translator, and tables for the most common breeds compare extra pounds on pets to extra pounds on humans, making it easier for owners to understand the significance of "a few extra pounds."

Benefits of Weight Loss Programs to Practices

Low Start-up Costs

The costs to the practice associated with starting a weight loss program are minimal.

- The hospital should already have floor or tabletop scales for dogs and baby scales for dogs and cats less than 30 lbs.
- Therapeutic diets designed for dog and cat weight loss are readily available and should already be in the hospital. Calorie densities for these foods are readily available (Tables 8.2 and 8.3).
- Useful tools are readily available. Pet food and some pharmaceutical companies provide body condition wall charts, tear-off score sheets, weight loss prescription pads, and client brochures free of charge.
- Start-up costs to announce, advertise, and educate clients about the program are minimal.

Table 8.2. Selected canine weight loss diets sorted by caloric density.

Products	kcal/100g DM
Hill's Prescription Diet® r/d, moist	298.4
Purina OM Overweight Management®, moist	300.5
Royal Canin Calorie Control CC 26™ High Fiber, dry	314.3
Purina OM Overweight Management®, dry	320.2
Hill's Prescription Diet® r/d, dry	325.4
Royal Canin Calorie Control CC 32™ High Protein, dry	354.1
Royal Canin Calorie Control CC™ High Fiber, moist	358.5
Iam's Veterinary Formula Restricted Calorie®, moist	389.8
Royal Canin Calorie Control CC™ High Protein, in gel	440.1

Table 8.3. Selected feline weight loss diets sorted by caloric density.

Products	kcal/100g DM
Hill's Prescription Diet® r/d, moist	316.9
Royal Canin Calorie Control CC™ High Fiber, dry	325.1
Hill's Prescription Diet® r/d, dry	325.8
Royal Canin Calorie Control CC™ High Protein, dry	349.5
Purina OM Overweight Management®, dry	349.7
Iam's Veterinary Formula Restricted Calorie, dry	360.3
OM Overweight Management, moist	366.1
Iam's Veterinary Formula Restricted Calorie, moist	389.8
Hill's Prescription Diet® m/d, moist	404.4
Royal Canin Calorie Control CC™ High Fiber, moist	412
Hill's Prescription Diet® m/d, dry	416.5
Royal Canin Calorie Control CC™ High Protein, in gel	428.1

Increased Revenue from Increased Compliance

The practice's increased revenue that results from increased compliance stems from:[20]

- Increased sales of therapeutic food
- Increased number of office visits
- Increased sales of products related to routine care (vaccines, flea and tick preventatives) not only for the overweight pet but also other pets in the same household
- Increased revenue from the early detection of diseases

Better Medicine

Pets that are seen more often at the hospital for weigh-ins and re-check visits are more likely to be vaccinated on time and receive flea and tick preventatives on a regular basis simply because the staff has greater opportunities to remind clients face to face. With increased visits to the clinic, concurrent diseases (diabetes, osteoarthritis, hypothyroidism) likely are better managed because of increased communication between the health care team and client. In addition, detection of late onset diseases (dental, cancer, cardiac, renal) may occur earlier in the progression than if the client only appears annually.

Summary

There are many ways to implement a weight management program. Pick the one that best complements the practice style and gain commitment from the entire health care team through education. By encouraging the health care team to lead by example, the benefits to the practice, staff, patients, and clients will be immeasurable. Maintaining a healthy body weight throughout life is perhaps the single most important aspect of increasing both the quality and quantity of life, both for people and pets.

In Practice

GO FETCH FITNESS™

Dr. Elizabeth Bixby of Taylor Veterinary Hospital in Cedar Falls, Iowa, has developed a unique weight loss program for people and pets, GO FETCH FITNESS™. This incremental walking program for a group of pets and pet lovers reinforces the relationship between pet owners and the veterinary health care team. It is a guide to help your clinic lead a six-week fitness and wellness education program to strengthen the bond between pet and owner and provide support and accountability among the participants. The program demonstrates to clients that the entire health care team is dedicated to enhancing and lengthening the relationship between people and pets through fitness and education. With GO FETCH FITNESS™, the client learns that her veterinarian is not only there to help in times of illness, but is there to promote wellness for her and their pet.

The GO FETCH FITNESS™ program can help your clinic be a proactive leader of preventative health care for your patients and your community. It is now available online (www.gofetchfitness.com) for use in your own clinic.

Busy Practice/No Time

The demands of professional and personal life often get in the way of implementing new ideas. Let's face it, change is hard; it is often easiest to continue the way we have always done things. But if you are frustrated with your current weight management program and don't think you have the time or resources to implement an effective program, Dr. Bixby's experience might just change your mind. The following is an account of why and how she developed GO FETCH FITNESS™ and why she is sharing this program with the veterinary profession.

Elizabeth Bixby: In Her Own Words

It was at the Iowa Veterinary Medical Association annual meeting that I first encountered Dr. Marty Becker and Dr. Robert Kushner's book, *Fitness Unleashed*.[14] The book suggested improving your health by

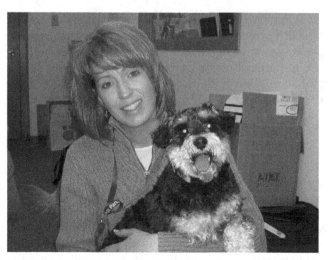

Figure 8.1. Dr. Bixby and Maisy. Photo courtesy of Dr. Bixby.

walking your dog and extolled the benefits that spending quality time with your dog and other dog lovers could bring. I wanted to start a group fitness program for dogs and people immediately. Then I got home. One of the kids was sick, school projects were due, instruments need to be practiced, I had a horse sale to work, it was my turn on call; the list went on and on. No exercise happened.

By the next spring meeting, the kids were a little older and I wasn't any thinner, or more importantly, any healthier and neither was Maisy, our Schnauzer. As luck would have it there it was, *Fitness Unleashed* lying on a table at the Hill's Pet Nutrition booth. I picked up a copy and was determined to carve out time for some type of fitness program at the clinic. In the beginning my motivation was selfish. The noon hour was the only 60 minutes of the day I could call my own. I searched the Internet for a fitness program for people and their dogs that would be educational and fun. Much to my dismay and surprise, I found nothing. I really wanted to copy and paste someone else's idea and hard work into our clinic. After all, I am a busy practitioner and mother. But I was also determined, so I decided to create a program of my own.

What exactly is GO FETCH FITNESS™? It is defined in the trademark application as a group fitness and education program for people and their dogs. The goals of the program are to provide dog lovers with information about nutrition, fitness, and a variety of pet-related topics; strengthen the bond between people and dogs; and facilitate friendships with dogs and dog lovers. The program provides accountability among participants. It also is designed to show the participants how much their entire veterinary health care team cares about them, their pet, and the special relationship they share. But the most important goal was to make all of this FUN!

Getting Started

I wanted the program to be an opportunity outside of the exam room to provide participants with valuable information about a variety of pet-related topics. I selected some topics from *Fitness Unleashed*[14]. Others are of seasonal relevance such as hot weather tips and hydration, and some were designed to help owners better understand disease processes (e.g., diabetes and hypertension). Additionally, I included a few topics (e.g., acupuncture) just because I have a personal interest.

I have a renewed appreciation for all of my teachers. Writing six weeks' worth of lesson plans was time-consuming and challenging, but being prepared paid off once the program got started. Having five young children, I found myself channeling Dr. Seuss. The result was the birth of a mascot, LuLu Lanigan. LuLu shares her thoughts and gives encouragement, usually in rhyme, throughout the program. For example, LuLu knows, "When you GO FETCH FITNESS™ for your dog and yourself, you will spend time together and retrieve your health!"

Key Point

When you GO FETCH FITNESS© for your dog and yourself, you will spend time together and retrieve your health!

Step 1

Choose a date and create a statement of "Official Details" for the program. One of the first calls I made was to our local YMCA. The director was excited to become involved with a community fitness program. Be creative; many local fitness or other wellness organizations are eager to get involved in community fitness programs and can provide valuable input for developing your program.

Our program is simple. Each group meets three times/week for one hour, and the session is six weeks. Our program met on Mondays, Wednesdays, and Fridays at noon. The initial meeting is dedicated to introductions and weigh-ins, followed by a short warm-up and walk. At subsequent meetings we start with a brief educational topic, then the warm up and walk. The walking time increases by five minutes each week, so the beginning discussion time decreases accordingly. Details of the topics covered in 2009 and 2010 are available at www.gofetchfitness.com.

Once you have the details, create a plan for promotion and advertising. Make a list of potential sponsors. Again, be creative; include both pet-related companies and local health-related businesses. I developed a standard sponsorship request letter and script for phone requests. It is important to be consistent when you are making so many new contacts. Don't forget to contact local government (city hall) if you plan to use parks or other open spaces.

Step 2

Develop a plan for distributing prizes and rewards. Create certificates of completion and assemble binders of information for the participants. The binders include outlines of all the discussions and any additional information you may want to include. This also is the time to create the area of your clinic that is dedicated to GO FETCH FITNESS™. Ideally, this area has a scale, posters, a team progress chart, and any other related information. During this stage you plan the walking route and order T-shirts and name tags. Useful tools that are available at www.taylorvet.com (Click on GoFetchFitness, then GFF Program Details) include a registration form with official details, registration information, prizes, great discounts, prerequisites, ways to participate off-site, a food diary, and an owner fitness progress log (Figures 8.2 to 8.5).

Step 3

Now is the time to get excited (if you haven't already!). Your hard work will soon be paying off. The immediate benefit of this program will be an opportunity to get to know your clients. Each group of people and pets will be unique, and the dynamics of the program will change based on the individual participants (human and dog). The motivation and perspectives differ for each participant. Having the time to gain an understanding of these motivations and perspectives through six weeks of class is what makes this program special. The relationships we create are the reason this program works. During the program most participants increase their physical activity and many lose weight, but the most important aspects appear to be the support the group provides. It is this sense of community that sets this program apart from other exercise programs.

The goals for GO FETCH FITNESS™ have expanded over time. We are now focusing our attention on obesity in school children. I have created two LuLu Lanigan children's stories and a GO FETCH FITNESS™ Kids Club song that are available for you to use in schools.

Recently I had the opportunity to visit my son's first grade class to share a new program called Go Fetch Kids™. I introduced myself with three titles: Mom, Mrs. Bixby, and Dr. Bixby, the veterinarian. I introduced myself this way because to a group of 7-year-olds, no one has more credibility than a married mom who happens to take care of pets.

The program involves a story, a song and of course some exercise. Well, as usual, the kids enlightened me. I led them through a series of questions and statements and asked them to shout out answers.

"We take our pets in to their doctor because we want them to be . . . "
"HEALTHY!"

"Why do we want our pets to stay healthy? Because we . . . "
"LOVE THEM!"

"We want our pets to stay healthy so they will live . . . "
"LONGER!!!"

Healthy, love them, longer. These were the unanimous answers from a group of 7-year-olds that perfectly describe this thing we refer to as "the bond." I see this bond daily when our 9-year-old spends a whole summer day making a new pillow and case of dog print fabric for the new bed for our pooch Maisy, and when our 4-year-old hugs Maisy around the neck and says, "Maisy doesn't want to go to work with you, Mommy. Her collar is bothering her today." When I look across our little camper strewn with a pile of five sleeping children and one very furry child fast asleep in the middle, I understand this bond.

These and many more are the reasons our clients seek out professional veterinary care. These are the reasons they bring their pets to us for a physical, vaccinations, and heartworm tests each year. These are also the reasons we as veterinarians must take the responsibility to teach our clients how to promote healthy bodies for themselves, their families, and their pets. The best way to support healthy pets and families is through regular exercise and proper nutrition.

Our pets add immeasurable value to our lives. We want them healthy because we love them, and because we love them we want them with us longer. GO FETCH FITNESS™ is one way we can foster and cultivate all of the special relationships that are created when a pet becomes part of a family. For more details please visit our website www.gofetchfitness.com.

GO FETCH FITNESS
Taylor Veterinary Hospital
Official Details 2010

WHAT: Go Fetch Fitness, sponsored by Taylor Veterinary Hospital and Blackhawk YMCA, is an exciting new fitness program designed to encourage people and their pets to exercise together.

There will be one six-week session with a maximum of 25 people and their dogs. Participants will be divided into small groups of three to four pairs (owner and dog) to make up a team. The teams will weigh in with their dogs on Mondays. The team results will be posted as a percentage of weight lost. Each team's progress will be tracked as the program advances.

The sessions will be held at noon and include daily educational discussions about human and animal nutrition and fitness followed by a group walking session that will be increase in time and intensity each week.

WHEN: **Go Fetch Fitness** will begin on Monday, April 12, 2010 and end on Friday, May 21, 2010. All teams will meet on Mondays, Wednesdays, and Fridays from 12:00 p.m. to 1:00 p.m..

WHERE: Teams will meet at Taylor Veterinary Hospital. This is located at 315 State Street, Cedar Falls, Iowa. Go Fetch Fitness participants will walk on a preplanned route along the Cedar Valley Trails.

REGISTRATION: Registration per session will be limited to 25 individuals and their dogs. One dog per registrant please. Participants may register at Family YMCA of Black Hawk County at 669 South Hackett in Waterloo, at Taylor Veterinary Hospital at 315 State Street in Cedar Falls, or they may print off a copy of the registration form from the

Figure 8.2. GO FETCH FITNESS© official details.

Taylor Veterinary Hospital website at www.taylorvet.com and drop it off at Taylor Veterinary Hospital before April 1, 2009 for the first session and before May 13, 2009 for the second session. The registration fee for each session is $20.00, which helps provide each participant with a copy of the book, FITNESS UNLEASHED for the first session if they have NOT already received one in a previous class, a Go Fetch Fitness t-shirt, and a variety of other fun incentive gifts.

WEIGH INS: Participants are encouraged to weigh in for their starting weight with their pet at the time they drop of their registration forms. The following weigh-ins will be on Mondays. Owners and pets may weigh in anytime between 8:30 a.m. and 5:00 p.m. on Mondays.

DEADLINES FOR REGISTRATION:
April 1, 2010

PRIZES: The team who shows the most improved fitness with the largest percentage of weight lost will win a year of free pet food for one dog from Hill's Science Diet pet food. Each member of the most improved team for each session will also win a free six-month membership to the YMCA.

PREREQUISITES: All dogs participating in the Go Fetch Fitness program must be up to date throughout the program on all vaccinations (distemper, parvo, bordetella and rabies), have a negative test for internal and external parasites and have identification tags or a microchip in case a pet should get away from an owner during a walk. NOTE: NO OUTWARDLY AGGRESSIVE DOGS WILL BE ALLOWED TO PARTICIPATE.

INCENTIVES: Taylor Veterinary Hospital will be offering special prices on microchipping and physical exams with vaccinations specifically for the Go Fetch Fitness program. Note that the regular price for microchipping a pet does NOT include registering that pet in a nation wide system.

Figure 8.2. *Continued*

This is usually an extra $19.00 that the owner pays to AVID, the microchip company. The incentive price below already includes this cost, which is a great savings.

Microchip regular price - $46.57   GFF price - $30.00

Annual exam *with* - $114.75   GFF price - $95.00
     Distemper, Rabies,
     Bordetella Vaccines
     and fecal exam

PART-DAY BOARDING: If you need part-day boarding to help work GFF into your schedule, you may call Taylor Veterinary Hospital. This service will be available to you at a reduced price IF space is available. We would love to pet-sit your dog, however we will have to give patients needing medical attention priority.

OFF-SITE PARTICIPATION: If you have a team of three to four individuals who would like to participate, but are unable to make it to Taylor Veterinary Hospital for the GFF group times, you may do so. The prerequisites and registration fees are the same and these participants will receive the book, t-shirt and gifts. These teams will need to send a representative periodically to pick up the weekly incentive gifts. The information discussed each day will be posted on our website (www.taylorvet.com).

CONTACT US: To acquire more Go Fetch Fitness program information, you may contact us:

        By telephone: (319) 277-1883
        Via e-mail: taylorvetrx@cfu.net
        Visit us on the web: taylorvet.com

Figure 8.2. *Continued*

TAYLOR VETERINARY HOSPITAL'S
GO FETCH FITNESS
REGISTRATION FORM

Session Dates: April 12, 2010 to May 21, 2010

Name: _____

Address: _____

_____

Phone Numbers: Home- _____

Cell- _____

Email- _____

Requested team members: _____

_____

_____

Pet's name: _____

Breed:_____

Age: _____   **Estimated weight:** _____lbs.

Sex: _____   **Spayed or Neutered:** yes or no

Vaccination History: Vaccinations <u>must</u> be current through May 21,2010.

Last date vaccinated for Distemper: _____

Bordetella: _____

Rabies: _____

Last date of negative fecal: _____

T-Shirt Sizes: ____ S ____ M ___L ___XL ____XXL

Registration Fee - $20 per participant x _____ = _____

Please make checks payable to Taylor Veterinary Hospital.

We encourage you to weigh in with your dog when you drop the registration form off. This will help minimize the time required to record initial weights.

Figure 8.3. GO FETCH FITNESS© registration waiver.

Go Fetch Fitness
Waiver and Release of Liability

Knowingly and at my own risk, I hereby register to participate in Go Fetch Fitness, and do hereby waive and release and forever discharge any and all claims, causes of action, demands and damages of any kind or nature that I, my successors or assigns may incur as a result of my participation in this event against Taylor Veterinary Hospital, T. James Taylor, Pamela L. Taylor, Black Hawk YMCA, the city of Cedar Falls, Iowa, the Cedar Trails system, and all sponsors, volunteers or any employees of these organizations for said injuries.

I further hereby certify that I have full knowledge of the risks involved in this event, and my dog and I are physically able to participate. I understand there will be no medical personnel on the walks. A good faith attempt will be made to contact 911 if an emergency situation arises. If as a result of our participation in Go Fetch Fitness, my dog or I require medical attention, I hereby give my consent to provide such medical care as is deemed necessary by emergency/medical/veterinary personnel.

I have no reason to believe my dog is a danger to other dogs or people. I hereby assume all liability for any injuries to any third parties caused by my dog. I understand that it is my responsibility to initiate and make financial arrangements for any medical care required for my dog as a result of my and his/her participation in Go Fetch Fitness.

I certify that I am familiar with the contents of this Waiver and Release, that I have read and understand the same, and that it is my intention by signing this Waiver and Release that the same be binding not only on me, but my heirs, administrators, executors, successors, and assigns. I hereby give my consent to let my dog and/or me be photographed for use by the YMCA and Taylor Veterinary Hospital in newspapers and other media for the purpose of publicity or advertisement.

Signature_____ Date_____
                  (Participant)

Figure 8.3. *Continued*

222

GO FETCH FITNESS PROGRESS LOG

My personal starting weight: _____
My dog's starting weight: _____
My teams starting weight: _____

My starting weight this week: _____
My dog's starting weight this week: _____
My teams starting weight this week: _____

Lifestyle and or diet mini-goals this week:

#1 _____
#2 _____
#3 _____

	Steps taken	Walking time	Personal/ Team notes
Mon.			
Tues.			
Wed.			
Thurs.			
Fri.			
Sat.			
Sun.			

Last weeks average steps: _____
This weeks average steps: _____
Week # _____

Figure 8.4. GO FETCH FITNESS© progress log.

GO FETCH FITNESS FOOD DIARY

	Breakfast	Lunch	Supper	Snacks	Notes
Mon.					
Tues.					
Wed.					
Thurs.					
Fri.					
Sat.					
Sun.					

Week #

Figure 8.5. GO FETCH FITNESS® food diary.

References

1. AAHA Leadership Addresses Major Association Projects. Press release: www.aaha.org, March 26, 2009.
2. Nestle M. 2007. Eating made simple. *Scientific American* September 60–69.
3. Radin MJ, Sharkey LC, Holycross BJ. 2009. Adipokines: A review of biological and analytical principles and an update in dogs, cats, and horses. *Vet Clin Pathol* 38:136–156.
4. German AJ, Holden SL, Bissot T, et al. 2009. A high protein high fibre diet improves weight loss in obese dogs. *Vet J* 183:294–297.
5. Bissot T, Servet E, Vidal S, et al. 2010. Novel dietary strategies can improve the outcome of weight loss programmes in obese client-owned cats. *J Feline Med Surg* 12:104–112.
6. Shay LE, Shobert JL, Seibert D, et al. 2009. Adult weight management: Translating research and guidelines into practice. *J Am Acad Nurse Pract* 21:197–206.
7. German AJ, Holden SL, Bissot T, et al. 2009. Use of starting condition score to estimate changes in body weight and composition during weight loss in obese dogs. *Res Vet Sci* 87:249–254.
8. Remillard RL. 2000. Clinical aspects of obesity management. *Compendium on Continuing Education for the Practicing Veterinarian* 23:29–32.
9. Cutt H, Giles-Corti B, Knuiman M, et al. 2007. Dog ownership, health and physical activity: A critical review of the literature. *Health Place* 13:261–272.
10. Kushner RF, Blatner DJ, Jewell DE, et al. 2006. The PPET Study: People and pets exercising together. *Obesity (Silver Spring)* 14:1762–1770.
11. Bland IM, Guthrie-Jones A, Taylor RD, et al. 2009. Dog obesity: Owner attitudes and behaviour. *Prev Vet Med* 92:333–340.
12. German AJ, Holden S, Bissot T, et al. 2008. Changes in body composition during weight loss in obese client-owned cats: Loss of lean tissue mass correlates with overall percentage of weight lost. *J Feline Med Surg* 10:452–459.
13. Zoran DL. 2009. Feline obesity: Recognition and management. *Compend Contin Educ Vet* 31:284–293.
14. Becker M, Kushner RF. 2006. *Fitness Unleashed*. New York: Three River Press.
15. Remillard RL. 2009. MSPCA Angell Animal Medical Center Pet Owner Survey: Feb 2008-Sept 2009.
16. Allan FJ, Pfeiffer DU, Jones BR, et al. 2000. A cross-sectional study of risk factors for obesity in cats in New Zealand. *Prev Vet Med* 46:183–196.
17. Colliard L, Paragon BM, Lemuet B, et al. 2009. Prevalence and risk factors of obesity in an urban population of healthy cats. *J Feline Med Surg* 11:135–140.

18. Kealy RD, Lawler DF, Ballam JM, et al. 2002. Effects of diet restriction on life span and age-related changes in dogs. *Journal of the American Veterinary Medical Association* 220:1315–1320.

19. Brice C. 2009. The biggest winners. *Trends Magazine* Jan./Feb. 45–47.

20. AAHA. 2003. The Compliance Equation. In: Grieve GA, Neuhoff KT, Thomas RM, et al., eds. *The Path to High-Quality Care: Practical Tips for Improving Compliance*. Denver, CO: American Animal Hospital Association.

Index

Practical Weight Management in Dogs and Cats, First Edition. Edited by Todd L. Towell.
© 2011 John Wiley and Sons, Inc. Published 2011 by John Wiley & Sons, Inc.

Randomized controlled clinical trial (RCCT), 89, 90f
Rat terrier, body fat of, 32f
RBW. *See* Relative body weight
RCCT. *See* Randomized controlled clinical trial
Relative body weight (RBW), 28–29, 29t
RER. *See* Resting energy requirement; Resting energy requirements
Resting energy requirement (RER), 67–70, 69t–70t
Resting energy requirements (RER), 37f, 38t–39t
Restricted calorie foods, 62–64, 63f, 64f
Retrieving, 150t
Rhodesian Ridgeback, 184t
Rottweiler
    muscle mass affects BCS with, 33, 33f
    standard weights for, 184t
Royal Canin Calorie Control CC™
    canine, 211t
    feline, 212t
Royal Canin Veterinary Diet™, 67t
    therapeutic weight loss foods for, 114t
Ruff Wear, 170t

Saint Bernard, 184t
Samoyed, 185t
Schipperke, 185t
Schnauzer, 184t, 185t
Scottish Deerhound, 184t
Scottish Terrier, 185t
Shih Tzu
    case study with, 42, 43f, 44
    standard weights for, 185t
Siamese cat
    standard weights for, 184t
    weight range comparison for, 28f
Siberian Husky, 185t
Silky Terrier, 186t
Single nucleotide polymorphism (SNP), 95
Slentrol®
    canine obesity management with, 135–38, 136f, 139t–141t, 141f, 142f

contraindications for, 143–44
dosing for, 135–38, 136f
    weight loss phase, 135, 136f
    weight management phase, 136–38, 136f
efficacy summary for, 137–38
percentage weight change in dogs treated with, 141f, 141t
precautions with, 143–44
study designs for, 139t–140t
warnings with, 143–44
Snausages®, 181t
SNP. *See* Single nucleotide polymorphism
Spaying, 108, 110f. *See also* Neutering
Staffordshire Bull Terrier, 185t
Static exercises, 150t, 159, 161f
Sussex Spaniel, 185t
Swimming, 150t, 160–62
Systems biology, 96f

Thera-paw, 170t
Therapeutic exercises, 149–70
    assessing and adjusting, 165–66
    benefits for dogs, 150t, 151–52
    cost and demands for dogs, 153–54
    dogs with medical conditions, 166–70
        obesity, 166–67
        orthopedic surgery, 169–70, 169f, 170t
        osteoarthritis, 167–68
    goals for dogs with, 149–50, 150t
    misconceptions with, 154–56, 155t
        dogs left out get exercise, 155–56, 155t
        dogs naturally know exercise, 155t, 156
        exercise is detrimental to arthritic dogs, 154, 155t
        exercise is traumatic, 154–55, 155t
        owners naturally know exercise, 155t, 156
    options for, 156–62
        Cavaletti rails, 150t, 161f
        fetching, 156
        mixed dynamic exercises, 160, 161f
        obstacle courses, 150t
        playing, 80–82, 156